DOES

Perspectives on the evaluation

IT

of HIV/AIDS health promotion

WORK?

Edited by:
Peter Aggleton
Andrea Young
Diane Moody
Mukesh Kapila
and Maryan Pye

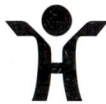

Health
Education
Authority

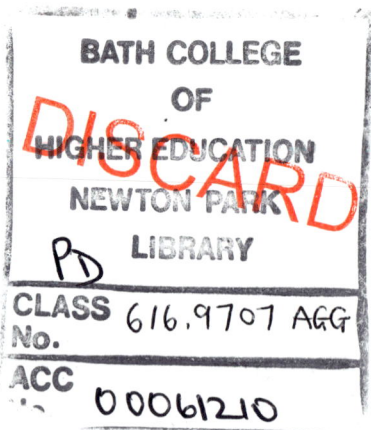

A CIP catalogue record for this book
is available from the British Library.

Published in 1992

Health Education Authority
Hamilton House
Mabledon Place
London WC1H 9TX

© Health Education Authority 1992

ISBN 1 85448 209 2

Typeset by Type Generation Ltd, London
Printed and bound in Great Britain by
Biddles Ltd, Guildford and King's Lynn

Contents

Introduction

This book has been produced as part of the Health Education Authority's strategy to support the monitoring and evaluation of local HIV/AIDS programmes. It brings together a range of papers given at a consultation on the evaluation of HIV/AIDS health promotion held at Bristol Polytechnic. Attending the meeting were evaluators and HIV/AIDS workers from health authorities, local authorities and voluntary agencies. The meeting provided an opportunity for experiences to be shared and for future training needs to be identified. The chapters that follow detail some of the different evaluation strategies that can be, and have been, used in work of this kind. We hope you find them relevant and interesting.

Peter Aggleton and Diane Moody
Bristol Polytechnic

Andrea Young, Mukesh Kapila and Maryan Pye
Health Education Authority

August 1991

CHAPTER ONE

Monitoring and Evaluating HIV/AIDS Health Education and Health Promotion

Peter Aggleton and Diane Moody

Evaluation is a term that is much used in health education and health promotion,[1] although there is no general agreement on what it means. To some, evaluation conjures up visions of elaborate studies in which one group of people is exposed to a new health education or health promotion campaign while another group is not. To others, it means pausing at the end of a training activity to think what went well and what went less successfully. To yet others, evaluation means handing out questionnaires at the end of a health education or health promotion workshop, analysing the data that comes back and writing reports. And to others still, evaluation is something which wastes time and detracts from the really important things that health educators and health promoters should be doing – enhancing the health and well-being of individuals and communities.

In work around HIV and AIDS there is also much talk of evaluation, and workers in local authorities, health authorities and voluntary organisations are increasingly being called on to evaluate and report on what they do. In some instances, evaluation is tied to future funding, with further support being conditional upon the success of present activities. On other occasions, it is linked to a concern to ensure that HIV/AIDS health education and health promotion activities 'work' – that they achieve what they set out to do. There are clear challenges here for HIV/AIDS workers, some of

1 There is considerable debate about the distinction between health education and health promotion. Health education encompasses many activities that are concerned not only with personal lifestyles but also with the social and environmental factors that affect health. Its focus is not just the general public, but also local and national policy-makers and health professionals (Whitehead, 1989). Health promotion, on the other hand, is generally understood as a broader term and includes all actions that improve health. These include a wide range of educational, political, legal, economic and social interventions to enhance well-being. Health education is therefore perhaps best understood as one component in health promotion. It is important to recognise that health education and health promotion are not unitary concepts and there are competing views about how each should take place (Tones *et al*, 1990). These views give rise to different styles or models of health education and health promotion, some of which are described by Aggleton and Homans (1987) and Aggleton (1989).

whom may lack the skills and expertise to be able to identify the most appropriate strategies by which to evaluate the activities with which they are involved.

This book describes some of the different approaches being used to monitor and evaluate local HIV/AIDS work in Britain. It examines a range of activities currently under way in health authorities, local authorities and voluntary organisations, and it points to some of the techniques that can be used to assess the progress and effectiveness of activities as diverse as staff training programmes, theatre in education projects, syringe and needle exchange schemes, and community development work involving men who have sex with men.[2] The book grew out of a consultation exercise, convened by the HEA, at which local HIV/AIDS workers and evaluators met to share their ideas, and at which the material contained in the following chapters was presented.

This introductory chapter sets the scene by offering an overview of some of the different ways in which monitoring and evaluation can take place. There is little consensus about the best way to evaluate health education and health promotion. On the one hand, there are those who favour a rigorous quantitative approach in which the emphasis is on measuring chosen outcomes and relating these to the interventions that have taken place. On the other hand, there are those who focus more qualitatively on the processes by which certain outcomes are brought about. Each of these emphases is associated with different research methods and, to the uninitiated, the choice can seem confusing. The aim in this chapter will be to demystify some of the terminology and concepts used in evaluation and to highlight the various techniques available. Subsequent chapters will demonstrate how particular approaches can be used and will discuss the strengths and limitations of different strategies. It is not the aim of this book to provide an authoritative guide to evaluation, more detailed guidance on this will be available elsewhere (Aggleton *et al*, 1992). The aim is rather to sketch out some of the key issues and areas of debate, so as to empower HIV/AIDS workers in their encounters with evaluation-minded colleagues and the relevant literature.

What is evaluation?

It is becoming conventional, particularly in the field of HIV/AIDS, to draw a distinction between *monitoring* and *evaluation* when it comes

---

2   Other publications produced as part of the HEA's efforts to support the monitoring and evaluation of local HIV/AIDS programmes include an edited collection of papers documenting the range and scope of local HIV/AIDS programmes (Pye *et al*, 1989) and three AIDS programme papers on the evaluation of HIV/AIDS health education and health promotion programmes (Pye and Kapila, 1990, 1991; Moody *et al*, 1991).

to looking at health education and health promotion programmes. The World Health Organisation (WHO) has recently defined monitoring as:

> the process of collecting and analysing information about the implementation of the programme: it involves regular checking to see whether programme activities are being carried out as planned so that problems can be discerned and dealt with.   (WHO, 1989)

Evaluation, on the other hand is best understood as:

> the process of collecting and analysing information about the effectiveness and impact of either particular phases of the programme or the programme as a whole. Evaluation also involves assessing programme achievements for the purpose of detecting and solving problems and planning for the future.   (WHO, 1989)

According to this approach, monitoring and evaluation are both important parts of the process by which the quality of HIV/AIDS health education and health promotion should be assessed. They are not clearly separable, except in so far as monitoring tends to concern itself more with the ongoing implementation of a programme, whereas evaluation concerns itself with the programme's effectiveness and impact. Other writers prefer to talk instead of two different kinds of evaluation – *outcome evaluation* and *process evaluation*. The former focuses on the extent to which the goals associated with a particular programme have been met, whereas the latter examines how they have been achieved.

Outcome evaluation

Many different kinds of outcomes can be assessed, including those that are *cognitive* (e.g. knowledge about HIV and its modes of transmission); those that are *attitudinal* (e.g. views about people with HIV/AIDS); and those that are *behavioural* (e.g. changes in personal or group behaviour). Important distinctions are sometimes drawn between *intended* and *unintended* outcomes (Eisner, 1979). For example, a number of HIV/AIDS health education and health promotion initiatives that intended to raise knowledge levels about the ways in which HIV is transmitted have also caused, as an unintended consequence, anxiety levels to rise. The kind of outcomes to be evaluated depends on the style of health education or health promotion adopted. Thus, work within an information-giving approach is likely to evaluate changes in knowledge and beliefs, whereas work which has a commitment to self-empowerment will evaluate the extent to which individuals feel more powerful after participating in the health education or health promotion programme. Similarly in the case of a community-oriented initiative, outcomes to be looked for might include the extent to which community awareness has been enhanced, the extent to which there was genuine community involvement in the project itself and the degree to which collective involvement in health issues is self-sustaining.[3]

Regardless of the kind of outcome evaluation being undertaken, reliable and valid *indicators* of what has been achieved are needed. An indicator is:

> an observable measure of the progress towards goals, objectives and performance targets   (WHO, 1989)

Within this framework, *goals* are general statements of programme intent (e.g. to modify behaviour patterns so as to reduce the incidence of HIV infection), *objectives* specify the desired end results of particular programme activities (e.g. the clients of sex workers will increase their use of condoms) and *performance targets* identify intermediate results contributing to the attainment of objectives (e.g. over the next six months, condom sales in urban bar areas will increase by 25%). An indicator, therefore, is something which indicates how much progress has been made towards a specified goal, objective or performance target. The majority of indicators aim to provide quantitative data on changes that have taken place (e.g. the percentage increase in syringes exchanged etc.). While some indicators may relate to the desired outcomes of a programme, the majority relate to intermediate goals, objectives or performance targets that will be achieved along the way. Illustrations of outcome evaluation can be found in the contributions to this book by Robert McEwan and Rajinder Bhopal (Chapter two), and by Graham Hart (Chapter seven).

Process evaluation

Process evaluation is very important in HIV/AIDS work since, without it, health educators and health promoters run the risk of identifying the outcomes of particular health education or health promotion activities without knowing how and why they were achieved. This is where process evaluation is important (Elliott, 1979). Process evaluation most usually focuses on the communication that takes place between health educators and health promoters and those they are working with. It examines the quality and nature of this communication by asking questions such as:

- Were health education messages presented in a culturally appropriate way?

---

3 For more details of what is meant here, see Homans and Aggleton (1988) and Aggleton (1989).

- Was the information supplied perceived as credible and relevant?
- Were the activities that took place threatening or involving?
- Was there a good match between the aims and intentions of the health educator and the needs of the clients?
- Were there group dynamics that interfered with the way in which health education messages were received and responded to?

The emphasis in process evaluation therefore is on studying the process of learning that takes place through health education and health promotion and on identifying factors that facilitate or impede individual and group behaviour change.

In contrast to outcome evaluation, much process evaluation is qualitative in nature since the emphasis is on describing the nature of the encounters that take place within health education and health promotion, rather than on more quantifiable outcomes. Examples of different kinds of process evaluation can be found in the chapters by Sue Scott (Chapter four) and Alan Prout (Chapter five).

Why evaluate?

There are several reasons why monitoring and evaluation can be important. First, they may enable health educators and health promoters to identify more clearly the consequences of their actions, be these short-term, mid-term or long-term, intended or otherwise, and measurable in terms of changes in behaviour or via other, more intermediate, indicators. Second, monitoring and evaluation can identify the processes by which particular outcomes are brought about. This way, health education and health promotion can become more transferable – not in an uncritical manner, but in the hope that the benefits that accrue in one context may do so in others. Third, monitoring and evaluation can enhance the accountability of service providers. It can indicate when perceived needs are being met, identify the factors that stopped a particular intervention bringing about desired goals, point to the alliances between different groups that led to successful outcomes and, in the final instance, aid decision-making about whether or not resources have been well allocated.

Some common evaluation strategies

There are, as HIV/AIDS workers will be only too aware, a bewildering number of strategies used in the evaluation of health education and health promotion. In this section we shall attempt to put these strategies into some sort of perspective by relating them to three broad approaches to the subject of evaluation.

The comparative approach

One of the most persuasive traditions in health education evaluation involves comparing two groups of people, one of which receives a special intervention or 'treatment' and the other which does not. The aim is to see whether this treatment has any special effect beyond that which might be produced by the passage of time. Treatments might include exposure to a new media campaign or participation in a new health education or health promotion activity (e.g. attending a new training workshop or going on an HIV/AIDS-related course).

The origins of this style of evaluation can be traced back to the research methods pioneered by agricultural botanists interested in evaluating the productivity of different seed strains and the effects of different fertilisers. By planting small plots side by side such that each plot varied to a known degree, botanists could get near to the controlled laboratory conditions advocated by chemists and physicists. Thus, variables (fertilisers as well as seed types) could be manipulated to discover those that produced the largest outputs. In health education research, clients may be given pre-tests (in much the same way that seedlings may be measured and weighed) and then submitted to different experiences or treatments. After a period of time, their attainment may be measured again to assess the effectiveness of the treatments they have received (Hamilton, 1976).

The group that receives the special treatment is usually called the *experimental group* whereas the group that does not is called the *control group*. Attainment may be measured by assessing changes in knowledge, attitudes and behaviour in the experimental group in comparison to the control group. In the simplest kind of experimental design (usually called a *true experimental design*), individuals are allocated at random to either the experimental group or the control group. Where this is not possible, and where the evaluator has little influence over how a health education or health promotion programme is implemented, a *comparison group design* may be used. This involves finding a group which is comparable in some way to the experimental group and examining changes in this group over time compared with those in the experimental group. For example, a group of teachers taking part in an HIV/AIDS training course might be compared with a group of teachers not taking part in the activity, after first matching the two groups for factors such as age, sex, length of service etc. Comparison group designs are not as strong as true experiments when it comes to identifying the causes of observed changes, but they provide a useful alternative strategy in circumstances where it is not possible to create an experimental and a control group (Figure 1).

Figure 1 **A before and after experimental design involving a comparison group**

Group	Pre-test	Receives activity	Post-test
Experimental	X	X	X
Comparison	X	–	X

When a suitable comparison group cannot be found, the group involved in a health promotion and health education activity can sometimes be used as its own control by taking the same measurements at intervals before and after the activity. This is called a *single group time series design*. Here, the success of the activity is measured by changes in the observed trend when the new activity is introduced, compared against baseline data collected earlier on. Such an approach might be used to evaluate the effectiveness of a local campaign publicising the existence of an AIDS helpline if the number and type of calls received over a period of months before a campaign commenced were compared with those that followed (Figure 2).

Figure 2 **A single group time series design**

Group	Test	Time intervals
Experimental	Pre-test 1	3 months before activity
	Pre-test 2	2 months before activity
	Pre-test 3	1 month before activity
		Activity
	Post-test 1	1 month after activity
	Post-test 2	2 months after activity
	Post-test 3	3 months after activity

While this kind of 'before and after' design is commonly used in evaluation, especially where there are limited time and resources, it is unfortunately one of the weakest approaches to use when it comes to identifying potential causes of change, since the question of what would happen without this activity cannot be answered. If this design is the only option available, it is important to look critically at the findings obtained before making claims about the effectiveness of the intervention.

There are several threats to validity in comparative evaluation. Some of these (known as *history effects*) may be due to other parallel events interfering with the interventions that have been made. For example, a national initiative which takes place alongside a local HIV/ AIDS health education activity may in fact cause the effects that the evaluator attributes to the local activity. The process of testing people may itself influence the results obtained, for example, by encouraging individuals to seek out further information on the issues discussed after the health education activity but before the post-test takes place. Finally, in some circumstances people may give the kind of responses they think evaluators want, particularly when questions are being asked about sensitive issues such as sexual behaviour and drug use. Care must be taken to train researchers appropriately so that this kind of *social desirability effect* can be kept to a minimum. Comparative styles of evaluation are examined by Robert McEwan and Rajinder Bhopal in Chapter two, and their application to the evaluation of syringe exchange schemes is discussed by Graham Hart in Chapter seven.

Objectives approach to evaluation

The origins of the objectives approach to evaluation date back to the 1930s in the United States when Ralph Tyler developed a style of educational testing that involved assessing the extent to which people attained the objectives that teachers and educators set (Tyler, 1942). During the 1950s, Benjamin S. Bloom developed Tyler's original work to come up with a classification system of objectives to cover most aspects of learning. Some of these objectives relate to *psychomotor skills*, some to *cognitive functions* and some to *attitudes and feelings*. Each of these three 'domains' can be subdivided. The cognitive domain, for example, divides the mental processes associated with learning into six categories: knowledge, comprehension, application, analysis, synthesis and evaluation (Bloom, 1956). Teachers and educators, it was believed, could be helped to evaluate their work if they specified in advance the objectives they hoped learners would attain. Data could subsequently be collected on the extent to which these had been accomplished. According to Tyler (1949):

> The process of evaluation is essentially the process of determining to what extent the educational objectives are actually being realised by the programme of curriculum and instruction. However, since educational objectives are essentially changes in human beings, that is, the objectives aimed at are to produce certain desirable changes in the behaviour patterns of the student, then evaluation is the

process of determining the degree to which these changes in behaviour are actually taking place.

Using this approach, evaluation involves:

- formulating objectives
- classifying objectives
- defining objectives in terms of behaviour
- identifying contexts where the achievement of objectives can be shown
- selecting promising evaluation methods
- developing and improving these methods
- devising ways of interpreting and using the results of evaluation.

(adapted from Jenkins, 1976)

In relation to HIV/AIDS health education and health promotion, this model implies that evaluation should be closely linked to the aims and objectives of specific programmes. If the emphasis is on changes in knowledge levels, for example, then these should be assessed in evaluation. And if the emphasis is on changes in attitudes, then these should be carefully examined after an initiative has occurred.

Face to face interviews and questionnaires are two of the most popular methods by which data can be collected in this style of evaluation, with questions being selected so as to relate either to the objectives of the programme as a whole or to specific components of it. Careful attention needs to be given to the selection of respondents from whom data will be collected, otherwise they may not be representative of the group as a whole. Selection can either be done *at random* or on a *non-probability* basis. Different kinds of non-probability sampling include *purposive sampling*, where selected individual respondents are chosen on the basis that they are 'typical' of the target group; *opportunistic sampling*, where the survey involves simply accessing all the members of the chosen group that can be reached; and *snowball sampling*, where key individuals are asked to suggest other people like themselves who might take part in the survey. This last kind of non-probability sampling could be used, for example, in a local survey of the effects of an HIV/AIDS health promotion activity on the attitudes and behaviour of injecting drug users. In the case of this group, no complete list of those who could be included in the study could possibly exist and, as a result, the most convenient way of reaching possible respondents is via an existing network of contacts.

Questionnaires and interview schedules will need to be carefully piloted before being administered to the group in question. Piloting should seek to eliminate ambiguities and to provide a realistic range of options in fixed-choice or 'closed' questions. It should also aim to ensure that the final product covers a sufficiently wide range of issues, produces reliable and valid data and is user-friendly.

While objectives-based approaches to evaluation cannot easily identify the *causes* of particular changes in knowledge, attitudes or behaviour, they can enable us to examine the relationship between the interventions health educators and health promoters make and the changes that do take place. This style of evaluation therefore offers a successful non-interventionist alternative to experiments, which may be impractical or unethical in many situations. Its use is discussed in the chapters by Robert McEwan and Rajinder Bhopal (Chapter two) and Wendy Clark (Chapter six) and, from a critical perspective, in Alan Prout's discussion (Chapter five) of the evaluation of community-based HIV/AIDS health promotion with men who have sex with men.

The interpretative approach

While comparative and objectives-based approaches to evaluation are the techniques most likely to be used in outcome evaluation, and while interviews and questionnaires may shed some light on the mechanisms by which particular outcomes are brought about, a more open-ended strategy is often needed when it comes to process evaluation. This alternative approach, which operates with principles derived from anthropology and interactionist sociology rather than botany or objectives-based curriculum theory, tries to identify how the various elements of a health education programme were perceived and understood by those involved. It thereby aims to *interpret* and *illuminate* how and why particular outcomes were brought about. Ethnographic research methods are the ones most often used in order to do this.

Ethnography is the study of culture, and generally involves researchers directly participating in the activity under investigation. The main ethnographic research technique is participant observation, and this involves either overt or covert participation in the situation under study. Good ethnographers are cautious about having too many preconceived ideas or hypotheses when they begin their work. Instead, they attempt to discover what is going on within the group that is under study. Ethnographic research therefore relies heavily on the quality of the researcher's involvement as well as on his or her observation and interviewing skills.

Interpretative styles of evaluation are likely to seek information from a variety of sources in an effort to identify competing perspectives on the processes involved. In the context of health education about HIV/AIDS, they often involve data collection from those who directly participated in a particular initiative, as well as those subsequently influenced by members of this initial group. Health promoters wishing to use this kind of evaluation technique may find it helpful to consider the kinds of data that should be collected in four critical contexts or environments – the professional context, the peer group context, the personal context and (for some) the parental context.

Several stages may be passed through when collecting and analysing ethnographic data. The evaluator's first concern is to become familiar with the day-to-day reality of the setting that is under study. Here, the evaluator may act like a social anthropologist or natural historian. For example, in carrying out an interpretative evaluation of an HIV/AIDS training course, it may first be necessary to gain familiarity with the ebb and flow of interaction, the principal participants, their attitudes and beliefs and so on. Having done this, attention may shift to a number of issues or topics for further, more focused, enquiry. Observation is then likely to become more directed, more selective and more systematic. Finally, efforts may be made to identify general principles underlying the organisation and operation of the course being studied. The aim here will be to spot possible patterns of cause and effect and to place individual observations within a broader context. Alternative explanations may need to be weighed in the light of the information gained (Parlett and Hamilton, 1972).

Naturally these different stages overlap and, as the transition is made from one to the next, issues become clarified and redefined. For example, what might initially be thought of as personal antagonism on a counselling training course may later be understood as conflict between different moral philosophies about safer sex. Similarly, what might first be understood as a lack of understanding on the part of a group of young people involved in an HIV/AIDS workshop may later be interpreted as a meaningful reaction to being confronted by culturally insensitive posters and pamphlets.

The course of this kind of evaluation cannot easily be charted in advance. But by beginning with an extended data base, and by progressively focusing on key issues, interpretative styles of evaluation can offer understanding and insight into the complex processes involved in HIV/AIDS health education and health promotion. While their in-depth nature may limit the amount of data that can be collected, and while the validity of these approaches is heavily dependent on the researcher's interpretation of the data, they hold the potential to identify more clearly the processes that led to effective outcomes, as well as those that led to less satisfactory consequences. A more extended discussion of some of the strengths of an interpretative approach can be found in Alan Prout's contribution (Chapter five) in this book while, from different perspectives, David Armstrong and Jean Hutton (Chapter three) and Sue Scott (Chapter four) demonstrate how this style of evaluation can be used with success in the evaluation of local HIV/AIDS programmes.

Thinking critically about evaluation

It would be inappropriate to end without some consideration of a number of 'difficult issues' in evaluation. These include questions of who should do the evaluation and to whom evaluation reports should be made available, as well as the uses to which evaluation findings should be put. In the space available here, we can do no more than highlight some of the considerations that need to be taken into account.

There continues to be much debate among HIV/AIDS workers about who is best placed to evaluate their work. On the one hand, the view is sometimes expressed that only those clearly associated with a programme will fully understand its aims and objectives, as well as the constraints under which it operates. On the other hand, there are frequent demands for external evaluation, since it is commonly supposed that this will somehow be more 'objective' and less tainted by the desire of health educators and health promoters to present their work in a good light. Both of these positions have their adherents and attempting some resolution between these viewpoints is no easy task. What can be said, however, is that evaluation is never a neutral and objective activity. Decisions have to be made about the programme elements to be focused on, the intermediate and output indicators to be examined, and also the aspects of the work that will not be evaluated because of lack of time and lack of money. And these decisions will be influenced as much by the prevailing moral, political and ideological climate as by the personal preferences of the evaluators themselves. The most important thing is for evaluators to identify clearly their position in relation to HIV/AIDS health education and health promotion, their past experience working in this field and the methodological approaches they favour.

In the majority of circumstances, a combination of internal and external evaluation may be the best approach to adopt, but this raises questions about the extent to which HIV/AIDS workers are adequately prepared to monitor and evaluate the programmes with which they are associated. Findings from a recent survey of local authorities, health districts and voluntary agencies suggest that many workers lack the confidence and skills to undertake this kind of activity (Moody *et al*, 1991). Training is therefore needed to help prepare them for the task. These same findings also raise questions about who might be best placed externally to evaluate HIV/AIDS health education and health promotion. Elsewhere in this book there is a spirited defence of the contribution that academics in higher education can make to work of this kind, and in health authorities there is strong pressure to apply the same systems of appraisal to HIV/AIDS health education and health promotion that are applied to other aspects of service provision. But to accept either of these options uncritically is to make the assumption that external evaluators are themselves adequately prepared for the work they will be required to undertake, and there is evidence to suggest that few are well versed in the complexities of local HIV/AIDS work. How many, for example, are aware of the different goals that can be aimed for in HIV/AIDS health education and health promotion? And how many understand why the pursuit of these goals may call for radically different strategies? Moreover, how many external evaluators can confidently say that they have critically examined their own attitudes to injecting drug use, and their own racism, heterosexism and homophobia (be these internalised or otherwise), to the extent of being able to identify the values they bring to their work and the interpretative biases that may result from these values? These are important questions to be asked by those contemplating commissioning external evaluation of their own work.

On the question of to whom evaluation reports should be made available, opinions differ. Clearly the needs of evaluation sponsors should be paramount, but participants in the evaluation process – paid workers, volunteers and clients – have interests too, as does the wider community of HIV/AIDS workers and health promotion specialists. Achieving a balance between the needs of these different groups can be challenging at times, as demonstrated by Sue Scott in Chapter four.

Evaluation findings are likely to be of greatest practical significance when evaluation is built into a project as an integral part of its design. That way, decisions can be made in advance about the policy and practice implications likely to emerge, and the means by which these can be made available to different stakeholders. This way too, planners and decision-makers can be alerted in advance to what an evaluation *cannot* tell them.

This book and the issues it addresses are likely to raise as many questions as they provide answers. This may be no bad thing, if in so doing they enhance the awareness of health educators and health promoters working in HIV/AIDS. As the UK epidemic enters a new phase, in which transmission between men who have sex with men is levelling off but where heterosexual transmission and transmission through injecting drug use continue to increase, this critical appreciation is much needed if effective interventions are to be identified. It is all the more important in a situation where efforts are being made to 'normalise' HIV/AIDS work and to render it accountable to the same institutional demands as other forms of health education and health promotion. It should not be forgotten that HIV/AIDS work encouraged health professionals of all kinds to engage with issues they rarely if ever addressed before – issues of discrimination against gay and bisexual men, issues of women's rights in relation to non-penetrative sex, issues to do with sex work, and issues to do with syringe and needle availability. And nor should it be forgotten that some of the most effective interventions in the field of HIV/AIDS have been those local and community-based initiatives so eschewed in the past by mainstream health education and health promotion.

References

Aggleton, P. (1989) Evaluating health education about AIDS. In P. J. Aggleton, G. Hart and P. Davies (Eds.) *AIDS: Social Representations, Social Practices*. Lewes, Falmer Press.

Aggleton, P. J. and Homans, H. (1987) *Educating about AIDS – a discussion document for Health Education Officers, Community Physicians, Health Advisers and others with Responsibility for Effective Education about AIDS*. Bristol, National Health Service Training Authority.

Aggleton, P. J., Moody, D. and Young, A. (1992) *Evaluating HIV/AIDS Health Promotion: A Resource for HIV/AIDS Health Promotion Workers in Statutory and Voluntary Organisations*. London, Health Education Authority.

Bloom, B. (1956) *Taxonomy of Educational Objectives. 1: Cognitive Domain*. London, Longman.

Eisner, E. W. (1979) *The Educational Imagination: On the Design and Evaluation of School Programmes*. New York, Macmillan.

Elliott, J. (1979) Curriculum evaluation and the classroom. Paper prepared for the DES Regional Course on Curriculum and Administration. Cambridge, Institute of Education, mimeo.

Hamilton, D. (1976) *Curriculum Evaluation*. London, Open Books.

Homans, H. and Aggleton, P. J. (1988) Health education, HIV infection and AIDS. In P. J. Aggleton and H. Homans (Eds.) *Social Aspects of AIDS*. Lewes, Falmer Press.

Jenkins, D. (1976) Six alternative models of curriculum evaluation. Unit 20, *Curriculum Design and Development (E203)*. Milton Keynes, Open University Press.

Moody, D., Aggleton, P. J., Kapila, M., Pye, M. and Young, A. (1991) Monitoring and evaluating local AIDS health promotion. *HIV/AIDS & Sexual Health Programme Paper 11*. London, Health Education Authority.

Parlett, M. and Hamilton, D. (1972) *Evaluation as Illumination: A New Approach to the Study of Innovatory Programmes*. Occasional Paper No. 9, Centre for Research in the Educational Sciences, University of Edinburgh.

Pye, M. and Kapila, M. (1990) Evaluation of AIDS health promotion programmes – concepts and the Cambridge study. *AIDS Programme Paper 7*. London, Health Education Authority.

Pye, M. and Kapila M. (1991) The story so far ... a review of the evaluation of local AIDS programmes. *HIV/AIDS & Sexual Health Programme Paper 9*. London, Health Education Authority.

Pye, M., Kapila M., Buckley, D. and Cunningham, D. (Eds.) (1989) *Responding to the AIDS Challenge: A Comparative Study of Local AIDS Programmes in the UK*. London, Health Education Authority/Longman.

Tones, K., Tilford, S. and Keeley Robinson, Y. (1990) *Health Education: Effectiveness and Efficiency*. London, Chapman and Hall.

Tyler, R. (1942) Purposes and procedures of the evaluation staff. In E. R. Smith and R. Tyler (Eds.) *Adventures in American Education Volume 3: Appraising and Recording Student Progress*. New York, Harper & Brothers.

Tyler, R. (1949) *Basic Principles in Curriculum Instruction*. Chicago, University of Chicago Press.

Whitehead, M. (1989) *Swimming Upstream: Trends and Prospects in Education for Health*. London, King's Fund Institute.

WHO, (1989) *Guide to Planning Health Promotion for AIDS Prevention and Control. WHO AIDS Series 5*. Geneva, World Health Organisation.

CHAPTER TWO

Context, Theory and Practice in Evaluating Preventive Health Education about HIV/AIDS

Robert McEwan and Rajinder Bhopal

Evaluations are constrained not solely by limits of time and money, but also by the beliefs and expectations of those who fund, undertake and participate in them. This chapter focuses on the impact of contextual factors on the evaluation of an HIV/AIDS-related theatre in education programme in the north of England. The initiative was funded by the Northern Regional Health Authority (NRHA), and was developed by a health education department in a district health authority. In this chapter we will examine how evaluation is deeply influenced by the context in which it takes place, the theory upon which it rests, and practical difficulties in its execution.

Context

In 1988, the regional medical officer (RMO) presented a paper to the NRHA proposing that young people were a high priority for preventive health education on HIV, and requested funds to support an educational programme. The NRHA supported the policy and provided funds. A multidisciplinary Working Party for AIDS Health Education was convened by the Regional Health Promotion Officer.

The working party was unable to identify a single effective method of AIDS education for young people and recommended that the funds be distributed to health authorities, on a competitive basis, for innovative projects. Further, it was recommended that funded projects be evaluated so that, in future, successful activities could be supported on a region-wide basis. Support for evaluation was therefore explicit in the regional strategy from the start.

In its report to the RMO, the Working Party for AIDS Health Education identified the overall aim and six specific objectives for educating young people about HIV; gave guidance on bidding for financial support for projects and listed six specific criteria for bids;

and identified ethical and controversial issues which it felt that projects should address. The overall aim was stated to be

> To develop, implement and *evaluate*, in the context of personal and social education, initiatives designed to minimise the spread of AIDS among young people in the Northern Region.

The NRHA supported 12 of the bids received in response to the working party's document. The Division of Community Medicine at the University of Newcastle upon Tyne was funded to support the initiative, through the synthesis and dissemination of information, cross-sectional surveys and evaluation. It was in this way that the authors' involvement with the programme began. Before looking in detail at one programme and its evaluation, the context in which these evaluations took place will be discussed.

Programme evaluation

The approach to evaluation advocated at the Division of Community Medicine at the University of Newcastle upon Tyne is influenced by many factors and naturally varies between evaluations. In all evaluations, however, the most important influence on the approach is the context in which evaluation takes place and, in particular, the people for whom the evaluation is undertaken. Three main interest groups can be identified. First, in 'participatory evaluations' the role of evaluators is to assist the powerless or oppressed to evaluate according to their own priorities (Rhaman, 1987). The objective is to correct imbalances of power between groups. Second, evaluations are often conducted for the sponsors or decision-makers in a programme, where the objective is to serve the interests of management and policy development. Third, the evaluator should seek to be fair and include the interests of other stakeholders affected by, or influencing, a programme e.g. academics, clients etc. (Lincoln and Guba, 1985).

These three groups often require different questions to be answered by evaluation, depending on their interests and the purposes evaluation serves for them. As sponsors and decision-makers, for example, district health authorities, for example, need evaluations to help manage programmes effectively, and to support bids for extended funding. The regional health authorities, on the other hand, need evaluation to develop and guide policy. Both of these agencies, however, have a vested interest in demonstrating the success of programmes. Academics, on the other hand, need to produce scientifically acceptable evaluations, to publish papers, and to appear politically neutral in interpreting results.

An influential factor in evaluation is the view of both the evaluators and evaluation users about what evaluation is and how it should be conducted. These perspectives on evaluation can be crudely classified in either *subjectivist* or *objectivist* terms. As Figure 3 illustrates, these philosophies imply contrasting views about reality, the objectives of evaluation, logical argument in evaluation, and the methods which can be used in evaluation.

Figure 3   Contrasting attributes of the subjectivist and objectivist approaches to evaluation

Subjectivist approach	ATTRIBUTE	Objectivist approach
	Reality	Stable
Dynamic		Universal
Individual		
	Objectives	
Gain		Seek out facts/
understanding		causes
	Logic	
Inductive		Deductive
	Methods	
Qualitative		Quantitative
Non-interventionist		Controlled
	Other features	
Empathic		Objective
Holistic		Particular
Non-generalisable		Generalisable

Some evaluators and evaluation users favour one of these approaches to evaluation, occasionally to the exclusion of the other. Health authorities, for example, generally favour the objectivist approach. This has important consequences for health education programme evaluators, as any use of the subjectivist approach must be backed by a thorough account of the adequacy and value of this approach. By combining, rather than compromising approaches, it may be possible to develop more comprehensive evaluations.

The potential and purpose of evaluation

After a programme has been introduced, evaluation can potentially address four sets of issues: the programme's implementation, its impact, its relative efficiency and its acceptability.

Implementation assessment has three purposes: to describe in detail the context, content and development of a programme; to establish as far as possible, the elements of a programme which lead to particular outcomes; and to monitor the achievement of organisational goals.

Impact assessment establishes the effects of a programme, particularly whether the programme meets pre-specified objectives.

Efficiency assessment establishes which of two or more programmes with the same objectives has the least costs and most benefits.

Acceptability assessment attempts to identify parts of a programme that are unacceptable to those who influence or are affected by the programme.

Few evaluations can include all of these aspects, because of resource constraints and programme features which limit the scope of evaluation. For example, a common problem is that impact assessment, using experimental designs, often cannot be undertaken because:

- programme objectives are not expressed in a suitable format for developing outcome measures
- this kind of assessment may not be considered ethically justifiable
- there may be too few participants
- there may be no suitable measurement instruments
- the costs may be judged to be too high.

It is rare for evaluators alone to determine the questions to be raised in evaluation and the purpose which evaluation will serve. These will usually be imposed by politically important stakeholders. Cronbach *et al* (1980) advises that, if evaluators are able to, they should seek guidance from clients, field-workers and policy-makers on the issues to be addressed in evaluation. All requests for information should be considered, but the final choice should exclude those questions about which there is least uncertainty; where study would promise little reduction in uncertainty; where the enquiry costs are high; and where the information produced would have little impact on policy choices or operating decisions.

In HIV/AIDS evaluation work in the Northern Region, efforts were made to include all four aspects in order to produce comprehensive programme evaluations. When technical or resource constraints forced a choice, the aim was to assess at least the implementation and impact of programmes. Nearly all of the 12 programmes funded by the NRHA sought ultimately to change the behaviour of young people and the aim was to assess the effectiveness of programmes in achieving their objectives. But quantitative impact studies in isolation may provide a narrow, and sometimes distorted, understanding of programme success and failure. Programme implementation was therefore examined in order to inform or explain the outcomes of impact assessment. Implementation assessment also provides descriptive information on the way in which the programme varies as it is implemented in different sites at different times.

Evaluation strategy

Once the subject of evaluation has been chosen, a research strategy is required to collect the relevant information. Strategies can include research designs such as experimental and cost-benefit designs. These designs in turn include methods such as randomised controlled trials, surveys or participant observation. Multiple designs and methods can be included in one strategy, and a single strategy may serve more than one evaluative purpose.

Ideally, a strategy should be chosen in consultation with evaluation users. Strategies which are not understood by evaluation users, or are against their prevailing philosophy, are unlikely to affect future policies or programme activities. Some strategies are appropriate for particular tasks in evaluation. For example, experimental designs using randomised controlled trials can be used to assess the impact of a programme. A 'stakeholder design', on the other hand, using qualitative methods, helps illuminate the understanding of programme implementation from the perspectives of clients, field-workers and managers.

Evaluation research strategies should ensure that information is collected in a disciplined manner. Smith (1981) describes how this may be achieved:

> For an enquiry to qualify as disciplined, it must be conducted and reported so that its logical argument can be carefully examined; it does not depend on surface plausibility, or the eloquence, status, or authority of its author; error is avoided; evidential test and verification are valued; the dispassionate search for truth is valued over ideology. Every piece of research or evaluation, whether naturalistic, experimental, survey, or historical must meet these standards to be considered disciplined.

Potentially, a wide range of quantitative and qualitative methods qualify as 'disciplined enquiry'. Evaluators using qualitative methods have different techniques for demonstrating that data are collected rigorously from those using quantitative methods. As Lincoln and

Guba (1986) write, qualitative data are gathered rigorously if it can be demonstrated that the data are authentic, fair and illuminative. Demonstrating rigour, however, usually refers to techniques to counter criticisms that the data may be inaccurate, non-generalisable or subjective. Both qualitative and quantitative research must be defended against these claims. Figure 4 details the different techniques used.

Figure 4   ***Quantitative and qualitative techniques to counter threats to rigour***

Qualitative solution	CRITICISM	Quantitative solution
	Something else explains what you have observed	
Prolong contact, observe continually, triangulate, check data with peers and respondents, analyse cases which disagree with your conclusions		Control sources of confounding by manipulating the experimental environment or randomise them between control and experimental groups
	Your findings relate only to those in your study or to one place or one time	
Describe in depth the programme context so that others may judge how applicable findings are for their context		Draw samples representatively, replicate the study in other sites and times
	Your own opinions have influenced the results	
Have a competent, disinterested external auditor check your data and interpretations		Separate the evaluator from the programme being observed and the people in the programme

(After Lincoln and Guba, 1986)

In the evaluation research carried out in NRHA, where the aim was systematically to gather information about a programme and its effects to serve the interests of policy development, programme planners and programme administrators, qualitative methods tended to be favoured for implementation assessment and quantitative methods for impact assessment.

Evaluating an HIV/AIDS theatre in education project

In order to show how these commitments informed practice, a recently completed programme evaluation will be considered. This concerned an HIV/AIDS theatre in education project. Data gathering is now complete in this evaluation, although the data remain to be analysed.

Theatre in education (TIE) first developed from the belief that drama can be used productively as a teaching medium. TIE programmes aim to explain facts and present arguments in an entertaining way, mixing theatrical forms and techniques with participatory education. According to Redington (1983), TIE is based on child learning theory and emulates the processes of early human learning by emphasising role play, simulation, problem-solving and empathy.

TIE programmes are usually run by actor/educator teams which tour schools and colleges, going through a pre-designed programme in each new setting. The programme evaluated here was a collaborative venture between North Tyneside District Health Authority and North Tyneside Local Education Authority, and was funded by the NRHA in April 1989. It included a play and drama workshop for young people aged between 16 and 19. In their proposal, the programme designers agreed to evaluate the programme. An informal meeting was held with the programme organisers in May 1989, at which preliminary thoughts about evaluation were discussed. The programme organisers stressed the importance of assessing implementation as well as the outcomes of the programme. In May 1989, a playwright was commissioned, and in June a steering group was set up.

At the first steering group meeting, evaluation was discussed broadly, although it was felt that its design would depend on issues raised in the play and workshop which were yet to be formulated. The second and third steering group meetings were held in September and November to discuss the script for the play. At the November meeting, development of the evaluation was again deferred as the content of the workshop had not yet been finalised. In December, a theatre company was appointed to stage the play, which was previewed in late January. At the preview, the contents of the parallel workshop were outlined. The programme was scheduled to begin in January 1990 and the final programme event was due to be staged in February.

Figure 5 represents the time-scale on which the programme and evaluation were planned and executed.

The programme

The play is set in the exercise room of a fitness studio in North Tyneside on one day in the autumn of 1989. The characters include

Figure 5 *The evaluation timetable*

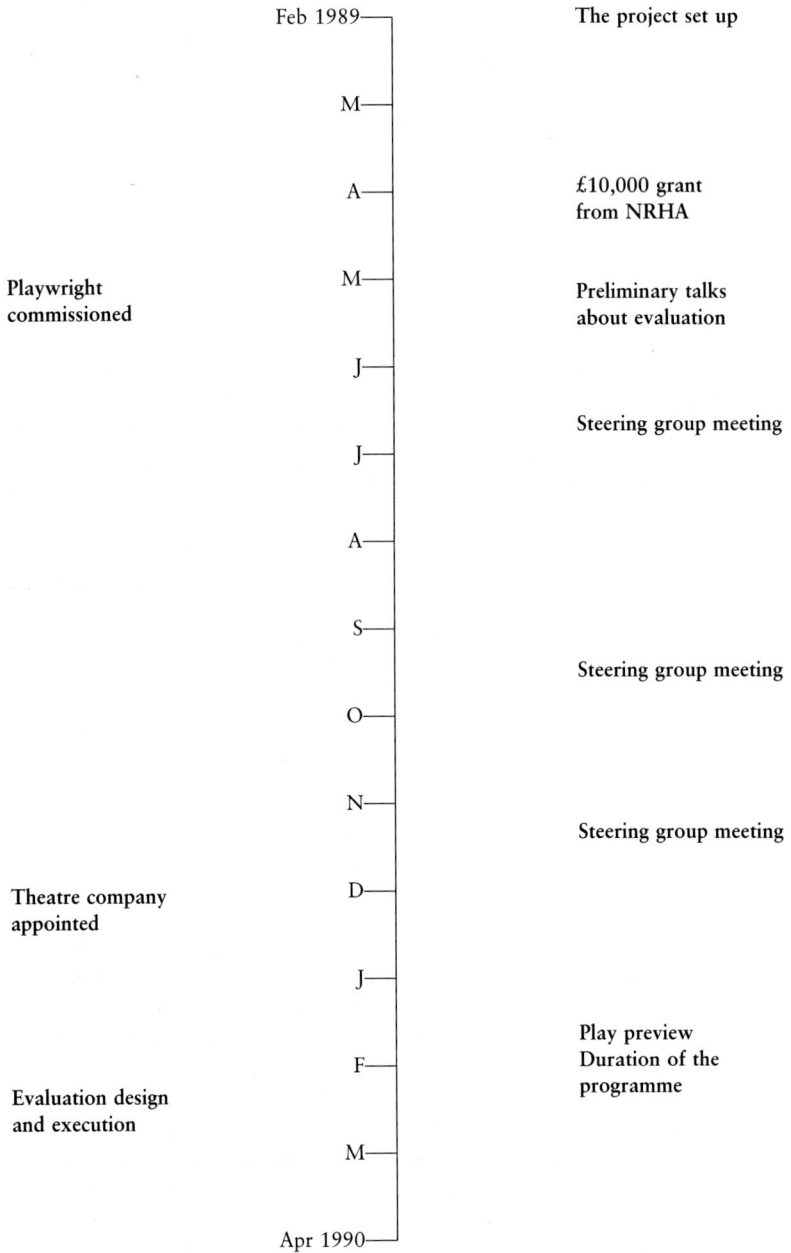

	Feb 1989	The project set up
	M	
	A	£10,000 grant from NRHA
Playwright commissioned	M	Preliminary talks about evaluation
	J	
	J	Steering group meeting
	A	
	S	Steering group meeting
	O	
	N	Steering group meeting
Theatre company appointed	D	
	J	
	F	Play preview Duration of the programme
Evaluation design and execution	M	
	Apr 1990	

Kirsty, a shy and impressionable 17-year-old Youth Training Scheme placement in the studio; Theresa, the worldly-wise manageress of the studio; Stuart, a clumsy, amusing painter and decorator; and Lee, an aggressive, macho fitness instructor. The play deals principally with Lee's deceit and infidelity in sleeping with both Theresa and Kirsty. This infidelity is revealed by Stuart, who inadvertently informs all three that Lee may have contracted HIV by virtue of a previous affair. As the 35-minute play ends, and Theresa and Kirsty realise they too may be HIV antibody positive, they ask each other, what are we going to do now?

A 45-minute workshop followed the play in which a maximum of 30 people could take part. The workshops, led by a Body Positive North East (BPNE) facilitator, included a hot seat session, role play, discussion and a question and answer session. In the hot seat session, participants anonymously wrote down on a card three things they would like to know about HIV. They also recorded one thing they would like to ask the characters in the play. Characters in role were asked a selection of these questions by the workshop facilitator. In the role play, and in five mixed sex groups, young people were asked about their thoughts and reactions at critical stages in relationships. Scenarios were provided; for example, on a first date a condom falls from the girl's handbag. Each group re-enacted such scenes in front of the other groups, with different participants offering their thoughts on the dialogue between the principal characters. Under the direction of the BPNE facilitator, the whole group then discussed each scenario and the reactions of participants to their situations. Finally, questions about the programme, and HIV-related issues in general, were answered by the BPNE facilitator. A graffiti board and display of posters and leaflets accompanied the programme.

Evaluation research strategy

A meeting was arranged with the programme organisers to discuss the evaluation of the programme in January 1990, on the day the programme was first staged. An evaluation research strategy was discussed and agreed with the programme organisers to assess the impact, implementation and acceptability of the programme using a variety of research designs. It was explained that assessing programme impact would meet the NRHA's needs from the evaluation. The programme organisers welcomed the offer to administer the impact assessment and collaborate on the design and execution of the implementation and acceptability assessment. The programme organisers were themselves experienced evaluators in the subjectivist tradition, and wanted to take part in the fieldwork for the implementation assessment, but, because of illness, were unable to do so.

Impact assessment

Two days after the programme was first staged, the programme objectives were reviewed. The intention here was to help programme organisers re-state the programme objectives in a format that was suitable for developing outcome measures. After lengthy discussion about the original programme objectives, the objectives the programme could realistically achieve and the effects which might be measurable, the following programme objectives were agreed: to personalise the risks of HIV infection, to promote self-determination with regard to sex, and to promote equal responsibility between the sexes with regard to safer sex and condoms in particular. The objectives of impact assessment were therefore to establish the effectiveness of the programme in:

- promoting self-determination and control in sexual relationships
- promoting equality between the sexes for safer sex
- personalising the risks of HIV infection.

To achieve these objectives, a pre-test/post-test survey design was used. The pre-test was administered one week before students took part in the programme. The post-test was administered immediately after the programme (see Figure 6). No suitable control group could however be recruited in the time available. Data were collected anonymously for this survey, although respondents were requested to record their dates of birth so that pre-test and post-test questionnaires could be matched.

The programme was to be staged in 26 schools, colleges and youth clubs, and one school and one college were selected for inclusion in the impact assessment, namely the school and college in which the programme was staged last. This allowed time for questionnaire design and for obtaining consent. In the college, students in the Faculty of Fashion, Tourism and Catering were selected, offering a potential sample of 200. The school offered a potential sample of 120 lower and upper sixth form pupils.

Table 1 **Response rates to the impact assessment surveys**

	Pre-test	Post-test
College (n=200)	115 (58%)	63 (32%)
School (n=120)	116 (97%)	89 (74%)

As Table 1 shows, the response rate to the questions was low, particularly in the college. While the administration of the questionnaires was supervised in the school, the college preferred to administer them via form tutors. A number of attempts were made to

Figure 6.   Sample questions from the post-test questionnaire used in the impact assessment

Q1   In general, how interesting are the following ways of raising AIDS issues for you?

	Very interesting	Quite interesting	Of slight interest	Not at all interesting	Don't know/ Not sure
Plays or dramas	☐	☐	☐	☐	☐
Written presentations such as leaflets	☐	☐	☐	☐	☐
Visual presentations such as posters	☐	☐	☐	☐	☐
Visual presentations such as videos	☐	☐	☐	☐	☐
Drama workshops (group discussions)	☐	☐	☐	☐	☐

Q14   How would you feel if a friend told you they had HIV? (Please tick a box for each statement)

	Yes	No	Don't know/ Not sure
I'd be disgusted	☐	☐	☐
I'd be sympathetic	☐	☐	☐
I'd feel lost and not know what to do or say	☐	☐	☐
I'd be worried for myself	☐	☐	☐
I'd rather they had not told me	☐	☐	☐
I wouldn't be able to believe it	☐	☐	☐
I'd want to stop seeing them	☐	☐	☐
I'd feel that I would not want to touch them	☐	☐	☐
I wouldn't want them in my home again	☐	☐	☐
I'd want to do my utmost to help them	☐	☐	☐
I wouldn't feel differently towards them	☐	☐	☐

Q15   How likely is it that you will do the following in future?

	Definitely will	Probably will	Probably will not	Definitely will not	Don't know/ Not sure
Avoid having a large number of sexual partners	☐	☐	☐	☐	☐
Keep to one partner only	☐	☐	☐	☐	☐
Avoid sex with people you do not know well	☐	☐	☐	☐	☐
Avoid sex altogether	☐	☐	☐	☐	☐

Q18   Have you filled in a questionnaire similar to this one before seeing the play 'Body Talk'?

Yes	No	Not sure
☐	☐	☐

Q19   Has watching this play caused you to think that you will change your behaviour in any way?

Yes	No	Not sure
☐	☐	☐

Q20   In your opinion, what messages was the play trying to get across?

_____
_____
_____

Q21   Were the messages of the play relevant to you and your lifestyle?

Yes	No	Not sure
☐	☐	☐

Q22   How interesting did you find the play?

Very interesting	Quite interesting	Of slight interest	Not at all interesting	Don't know/ Not sure
☐	☐	☐	☐	☐

increase the response rate in the college, but with limited success. Data from the survey are being analysed using the Statistical Package for Social Sciences (SPSS) computer software.

Implementation assessment

The objectives of implementation assessment were to describe:

- the programme and its effects from the perspectives of young people
- the programme in different sites
- how the programme developed over time.

Two methods were used to achieve these objectives – non-participant observation and focused group discussions. To complement information obtained in this way, programme organisers kept a record of organisational developments over time.

The objectives of the non-participant observation were to describe:

- programme activities in different sites
- the physical and social environment in which the programme took place
- the reactions of participants to programme events.

Observational data were recorded in a notebook, and notes were later rewritten. The programme was observed in one school and one college. Data from observation are to be transcribed and analysed using HYPERSOFT, a software package for analysing text based data-sets.

The objectives of the focused group discussions were:

- to describe programme activities from the perspectives of young people
- to describe participants' expectations of the programme
- to discuss the objectives of the programme
- to discuss the programme's effects on participants
- to discuss the suitability of the programme for other groups.

After the programme organisers and the writers had identified the objectives for implementation assessment, an extensive aide-memoire of topics for discussion was drawn up jointly. This aide-memoire was further refined by cutting out topics of least interest before the first discussion was held. The topics for discussion were later developed to explore issues raised in previous discussions. With the consent of groups, discussions were tape-recorded.

A sampling strategy for the discussions was discussed with programme organisers. This was developed from the work of Patton (1987), and involved three discussions with mixed sex groups of approximately eight young people. The three groups were an older group of college students (aged 18 or 19) who had seen the play only, a younger group of school pupils (all aged 16) who had taken part in workshops, and a mixed group of college students (aged between 16 and 18), some of whom had not taken part in workshops. Tape

Figure 7 **Aide-memoire for focused group discussion**

Prompts for discussion: the play

What did you expect before you saw the play?
What were the messages of the play?
Were these messages relevant to you?
What age group is the play suitable for?
What were your feelings throughout the play?
What was your main feeling at the end of the play?
Were the characters in the play like you in any way?
Were the characters like anybody you know?
Can watching plays change your opinion about something?
Did this play make you think differently about anything?
Was the play worthwhile watching?
Was it entertaining?

Prompts for the discussion: the workshop

How were you selected to take part in the workshop?
Why did you volunteer?
What did you think the workshop was going to be about?
What happened in the workshop?
Why were these activities undertaken?
Should the workshop be mixed or single sex?
What age group should take part in the workshop?

recordings are being transcribed for analysis with the help of HYPERSOFT. Analysis will be undertaken by programme organisers as well as the authors.

Acceptability assessment

The objectives of acceptability assessment were:

- to establish the interest and entertainment value of the programme
- to describe and assess the level of anxiety generated by the programme.

To achieve these objectives, data collection techniques similar to those employed in the implementation and impact assessments were used. In the implementation assessment, participants' emotional reactions to the play and workshop were observed. Students' feelings before, during and after the programme were identified by group discussions. Additionally, participants were here asked to review the best and worst parts of the programme. In the impact assessment, pre-test ratings of different educational strategies, including TIE, were obtained. Anxiety about HIV was also assessed before and after the respondents took part in the programme, by asking respondents to rate how worried they were about HIV, how likely they were to know someone with HIV in their lifetime, and whether they felt personally at risk from HIV.

Findings and implications

Results from this evaluation will be reported to and discussed with young people who took part in it, the establishments in which evaluation took place, and the district and regional health authorities. One purpose of reporting results back to young people and programme organisers is to check on the reliability of interpretations. Additionally, the establishments concerned will be interested to learn whether such programmes are educationally valuable. The district health authority might use the results of evaluation to develop future TIE programmes, or to apply for funding to extend the current programme if it is found to be successful. Finally, the NRHA will use the evaluation to help influence decisions about whether such programmes should be supported elsewhere in the region.

An important contextual influence on this evaluation was the control of its planning and execution. Throughout the course of the work, it became apparent that both the programme organisers and the writers believed that the others held responsibility for the evaluation. It was unclear what would be the appropriate level of external involvement required to ensure that programmes were effectively evaluated. Clearly, this would vary between programmes, but early thoughts indicated that advice would be given only on evaluation. It transpired that the programme organisers wanted and expected us to evaluate the programme, but were unaware of the time we would need to design and execute an effective evaluation. At the same time, we were unaware that the programme was at such an advanced stage without any firm plans for evaluation.

Effectively, the evaluation was designed, organised and executed within a period of three weeks, which constrained what could be achieved in a number of ways. First, the evaluators 'took over' the evaluation more than they hoped would have been necessary. Second, the evaluation had to be carried out in the chosen establishments, even though in one establishment the evaluators had no control over how the impact assessment questionnaires were administered. Third, manpower constraints limited the ability to carry out group discussions and observe the programme in different settings in the time available. Although its execution was rushed, the evaluation has, however, produced useful data on which this TIE programme may be judged, particularly in schools. Initial data suggests that the programme has been successfully implemented, and to good effect.

Programme organisers were asked to comment on this chapter. The following is their written response.

> We remain as convinced as we were at the outset of the value of evaluation in programme design. We found the offer of help from the University most welcome, and for this reason, we sought to involve the evaluator in our planning and discussions from an early stage. Our understanding was that we had been offered practical help and support by the University Department of Community Medicine and that they were offering their expertise, resources and experience to provide an effective and meaningful evaluation process.
>
> Although both the authors were familiar with the different possible approaches in evaluation and had strong opinions on the type of approach best suited to the objectives of this project, neither had extensive experience in formal evaluation procedures and both lacked awareness of, for example, the time-scale necessary to set up and implement evaluation of the type required.
>
> Neither had experienced the use of an external agency in implementation and design. Consequently the authors were not aware of the different perspectives of different stakeholders, nor did they feel that reconciling these was their responsibility. While they accept that in the event the time-scale in which to set up the evaluation was left unrealistically short, they feel that they are not entirely responsible for this and that failure of the evaluator to alert them to this possibility contributed at least in part to what happened subsequently.
>
> Using the University as an external evaluator has many attractions and potential benefits for programme organisers. However, it is important to clarify from the outset the role the external evaluator will play in the entire process, otherwise confusion can arise, different expectations and assumptions can emerge and differing needs from evaluation remain hidden. Any of these problems can work against a successful outcome and mar a potentially fruitful relationship. We hope that the lessons we have learned from this exercise will enable others to avoid such pitfalls in future and look forward to the next opportunity to work in this way when we can put the lessons into practice.

Conclusions

Experience of assisting in the evaluation of preventive health education programmes suggests some general principles about how such evaluations can be better organised. The resource requirements for evaluation must be clearly identified when innovative programmes are proposed. Funding agencies and programme organisers need to be aware of how much work evaluation entails. Those unaccustomed to evaluation may underestimate what is entailed here.

Ownership or responsibility for an evaluation needs to be agreed at an early stage. It is then the responsibility of the evaluator to understand the interests of major stakeholders in an evaluation, and to communicate each stakeholder's interests to others. The evaluator should seek to represent the various interests in an evaluation and, where possible, to base the evaluation on their ideas about what evaluation is and how it should be conducted.

Some health educators may have little interest or experience of evaluation or have an interest but be overwhelmed by the organisational demands of implementing a programme. In these circumstances, superficial evaluations may result. These may not meet the requirements of principal stakeholders in the programme. Early agreement between stakeholders on an acceptable evaluation and an evaluation timetable should help to avoid this problem. While some health educators are experienced evaluators, many need training concerning the role and scope of evaluation, its benefits and shortcomings, on how to commission an evaluation, and on how to use evaluation results. Those health educators who wish to carry out programme evaluations themselves may need training. They may also need support and advice on technical research matters such as sampling or statistical techniques. Finally, the non-specialist evaluator needs access to the tools of the professional researcher. For example, computing facilities will usually be required, and audio-visual and tape-recording equipment will be needed occasionally.

The importance of rigorous evaluation of preventive health education about HIV/AIDS is clear. Without it, we cannot be sure which strategies are most effective in restricting the spread of HIV infection. Because trained evaluators remain in short supply in the health service, health educators will need to undertake evaluation themselves. The NRHA, through sponsoring the project, has ensured that the innovative educational programmes in its region are being evaluated. Through collaborative work, the project hopes to enhance the training of health educators so that in future they can evaluate their own work, with the minimum amount of external guidance and technical assistance.

Acknowledgements

Our thanks to Wendy Patton and Ian Atkinson of North Tyneside District Health Authority and Local Education Authority respectively, for their help and advice in writing this paper. Thanks also to the NRHA for sponsoring our project. Lastly, we thank Kate Warren for clerical, secretarial and moral support in all of our work.

References

Cronbach, L.J. *et al* (1980) *Towards Reform of Program Evaluation.* San Francisco, Jossey Bass Publishers.

Lincoln, Y.S. and Guba, E.G. (1985) *Naturalistic Inquiry.* Beverly Hills, Sage.

Lincoln, Y.S and Guba, E.G. (1986) Trustworthiness and authenticity in naturalistic evaluation. In D.D. Williams (Ed.) *Naturalistic Evaluation.* San Francisco, Jossey Bass Publishers.

Patton, M.Q. (1987) *How to use Qualitative Methods in Evaluation.* Beverly Hills, Sage.

Redington, C. (1983) *Can Theatre Teach?* Oxford, Pergamon Press.

Rhaman, M.A. (1987) The theory and practice of participatory action research. In J.R. Shadish and C.S. Reichardt (Eds.) *Evaluation Studies Annual Review,* Volume 12. Beverly Hills, Sage.

Smith, M.L. (1981) Naturalistic research. *Personnel and Guidance Journal* 59, 586.

CHAPTER THREE

A Systemic Model for Evaluating Local HIV/AIDS Health Promotion Programmes[1]

David Armstrong and Jean Hutton

The Cambridge AIDS Programme was set up by the Cambridge Health Authority in 1987 on a budget of £120,000. It evolved out of, and brought together, a variety of local statutory and voluntary initiatives in the field of health promotion and health education, in which individuals from the Authority had taken a leading and supportive role. The Programme comprised four core elements:

- a voluntary AIDS Helpline with back-up services operating from its own premises in the city
- a needle exchange linked with counselling and advice from two drugs agencies
- an HIV testing, counselling and advice service from the genito-urinary medicine clinic at Addenbrooke's Hospital
- an AIDS Education Unit offering training, information and consultancy within the Authority and to local agencies and organisations.

The first three of these core elements were already in existence and were organisationally independent of the Programme. The fourth element (the AIDS Education Unit) was set up under the Programme with a team manager, two trainers and an administrator, as the major training and consultancy resource for the Programme's work with agencies in the community.

Leadership of the Programme was vested in a director who had

---

1. *Editor's note*. Local HIV/AIDS health promotion can be seen as a series of discrete, apparently independent activities. More often there is an attempt to provide a co-ordinated programme which links individuals, groups and organisations throughout the community in a wide range of complementary activities. Evaluation of this work may concentrate on individual projects, or may examine the processes by which health promotion activity is enabled and enacted. The model of evaluation described here adopts this latter approach and was generated from an evaluation of the Cambridge AIDS Programme carried out by The Grubb Institute for the Cambridge Health Authority and the Health Education Authority in 1988.

been, from her previous position as sister in the genito-urinary medicine clinic, a prime mover in promoting voluntary and statutory initiatives in HIV/AIDS health promotion in Cambridge. She was well known to staff and workers associated with each of the pre-existing core elements, and the conception and creation of the Programme reflected ideas and proposals with which she had been closely associated throughout.

As director, her stated responsibilities were 'to support, co-ordinate and take [the four elements] forward, ensuring that they cross-refer and train each other as well as ensuring that they have the resources they need to continue'. Effectively, it was the director therefore who shaped the strategy on which the Programme as a whole operated: liaising with an advisory group set up under the Joint Consultative Committee structure and with regional bodies; promoting the work of the Programme in the community and its agencies; and sustaining and developing its distinctive philosophy and approach. The director reported directly to the chief executive of the Authority through a small steering committee chaired by him: a decision which reflected a deliberate intention to establish the Programme within the Authority, but independent of its existing departments and structures. Within this structure, the Programme worked with agencies, organisations, community groups and individuals across the Cambridge Health District. The district has a population of approximately 270,000 with a significant transient population of young people from the UK and overseas. The known incidence of HIV/AIDS in the district and in the region was low. However, the high concentration of young people, the Authority's and the University's reputation in HIV/AIDS research, and less tangible factors associated with the culture of the community all contributed to sustain levels of interest and concern in the community's response to HIV/AIDS. The Programme was therefore strategically placed to focus on and work with this response.

Organisational evaluation

Evaluation of any programme, in this field as elsewhere, will always be relative to particular purposes: of the sponsors, organisers, staff, stakeholders or others. There is no generic model of evaluation applicable to each and every case. Evaluation is also a powerful intervention in the activities of a programme, requiring access to people, records and documentation. Unless there is some clarity, agreement and ownership about what is being evaluated, and why and how, there are likely to be unanticipated consequences which will affect the quality and reliability of the work and/or its subsequent use.

In this case, the need for some evaluation of its work was recognised by the Cambridge AIDS Programme from the beginning and actively canvassed by the director. Evaluation was seen to be important because the Programme represented a significant investment of a local health authority's resources in a field of national significance. It also offered a new, innovative and untried organisational approach to health promotion in the field of HIV/AIDS. The reference here to organisational approach is important. While evaluative studies of particular methods or techniques of health promotion and/or health education are not uncommon, less attention has been paid to organisational initiatives and their management and to the ways in which these support, develop, extend and diffuse effective practice within a community and its agencies. It was this aspect that was at the centre of the Programme's concern.

It was anticipated that evaluating the Programme and its work could contribute new insights into community-based approaches to HIV/AIDS health promotion and establish what makes for effective self-generating interventions in community responses to HIV/AIDS. The evaluation process looked to identify strengths and weaknesses in the programme structure, strategies and methods, to provide a basis for reviewing policy, organisation and resourcing, and to support staff learning and innovation. Overall, it was intended to provide a qualitative measure of return on investment.

While some of these purposes were specific to this particular programme in its context, it was recognised that what emerged from the evaluation might have a wider significance for similar initiatives undertaken elsewhere. With this in mind, the Programme director approached the Health Education Authority for support in undertaking an independent evaluation study. The proposal fitted into the HEA's own programme of seeking to sponsor evaluative studies in this field, but it in turn added an additional element. This was that the proposed evaluation should also seek to develop an approach to the evaluation of organisational initiatives at a local level which was capable of replication, either externally or in-house. While this last element clearly needed to be borne in mind throughout the evaluation, it did not significantly affect the way the evaluators worked with the Programme and its staff. The model of evaluation outlined below evolved continuously throughout the study and as presented here is probably somewhat tidier than it appeared at the time.

Initial discussions were held with the evaluation steering group which included representatives of the Programme, Cambridge Health Authority and the HEA. The task of evaluation was initially defined as

- to find out the difference the Programme was making to how communities and agencies in Cambridge were relating to the realities of HIV infection and AIDS
- to identify the factors which contributed to this difference

- to enable those responsible for the Programme and others to assess the implications for policy, resourcing and future operations in respect of this Programme and also of similar initiatives undertaken elsewhere.

As the evaluation proceeded, however, it became necessary to reformulate this initial statement of aim in a way which more precisely reflected the realities and experience of evaluation – i.e.

to establish the grounds for organisers and sponsors to assess the relevance and effectiveness of the Programme for the needs of the local community.

The method identified to achieve this aim was:

to investigate the activities of the Programme so as to identify their outputs (defined as the difference made by the Programme's activities to the beliefs, attitudes and practices of members of the community and its agencies) and to relate these to the intentions, values and resources of the organisers, within the geographical, social, political, economic and health contexts of the Programme itself.

This reformulation acknowledged that at present any programme operating in this field has to work as much, if not more, with the not-known as with the known. The area of work is new and innovative. HIV infection and AIDS are a major threat, actual and potential, to the health of the community. They arouse fear and anxiety. The human and social implications are far-reaching, affecting relations between members of the community and its agencies in unpredictable ways. There are no tested models of how best to meet this challenge, and organisers of programmes necessarily have to take risks and act on judgements which cannot always be objectively supported, at least in the short run. Yet they and their sponsors need some basis on which they can be realistically confident in what they are doing. This requires the capability of being alert to the judgements and assumptions they are making and of looking for evidence to test these and adapt or change them where needed. In such a context, evaluation is essentially an action-research tool: a method for comprehending and illuminating what is happening in a way which will inform judgements and decisions at every level.

A systemic approach

The systemic approach to evaluation described here is not the only approach to evaluation, nor is it necessarily the appropriate approach in other circumstances. It is, however, a strategy which fits the realities and concerns which those undertaking organisational initiatives in this field currently face. A systemic approach seeks:

- to identify and understand the boundaries around the activities of the programme – boundaries of task, technology and time
- to comprehend the programme as a system, both in respect of its aims and in respect of what is actually happening
- to focus both on outputs and on processes
- to generate information rather than to collect data
- to interpret and not simply describe.

There are two further implications of a systemic approach to be considered. First, attention is continually being focused on the connections between what is happening in different parts or elements of a programme, and how this is reflecting, overtly or covertly, the programme's relation to its context. The programme is thereby seen holistically, rather than as a sum of several discrete activities. Second, in this approach, apparent areas of difficulty or problems are not primarily interpreted at their face value as evidence of some dysfunction. Instead, they are seen in relation to how the programme as a whole functions in its context. Thus the key question evaluators need to be alert to is not 'Why is this happening?' but rather 'If this is happening, why does it need to be happening?' Unless this question is kept continually in mind there is a real risk of making premature and piecemeal judgements.

The model evolved during the study comprised five overlapping, sequential stages. Each stage can be identified by a particular aim and method, as set out in Table 2 below. A fuller account of the five stages, the particular instruments designed and used and the findings relating to the Cambridge AIDS Programme has already been published by the HEA (Pye and Kapila, 1990). Here, some of the conceptual and methodological considerations underlying the model and its practical application will be considered.

Stage 1: The need for system description

It can be argued that evaluation of any planned organisational initiative must start from some analysis of that initiative understood as a system (i.e. activities with a boundary), interacting with its environment to do something, produce something, or bring about or contribute to some planned or desired change. This analysis, however, cannot simply be read off current documentation about intended activities, resources, structures and aims.

In the case of new and innovatory ventures, for example, the

Table 2 **The five stages of systemic evaluation**

Stage 1

System description

Aim	To establish:
	The organisational model which best fits how the programme is operating and being managed.
	The statement of aim which best corresponds to what the programme is actually working to achieve.
Method	To examine current documentation and to interview representatives of the programme on how they understand the programme and its activities.
	To formulate a working description of the programme and its aim.
	To test this description with the programme organisers and make adjustments as needed.

Stage 2

Identifying performance indicators

Aim	To determine and agree indicators for assessing how what is happening in the programme is contributing to the achievement of its aims.
Method	To use material gained from Stage 1 to identify specific, realistic and appropriate measures of performance.
	To design an evaluation profile based on indicators to be used in assessing performance, and relevant sources and methods for gathering data.
	To agree this with the programme organisers.

	Stage 3

Generating information on programme operations and performance

Aim	To use the indicators to collect and interrogate data on all the operations of the programme.
Method	To design specific instruments for collecting and processing data on programme operations based on the evaluation profile (Stage 2).
	To organise and carry out fieldwork, through eg:
	Focus group discussions Interviews Activity analysis Participant observation of courses/meetings Scrutiny of records Utilisation of existing local research Surveys Media analysis – coverage and content.

	Stage 4

Matching findings to system description

Aim	To assess the programme's effectiveness in relation to the description of the programme and its aim.
Method	To analyse and interpret the findings from Stage 3.
	To test how far they confirm or modify the stated description of the programme and its aim.

Stage 5

Implications for programme policy and operations

Aim   To provide a basis on which programme organisers and staff can make decisions about the development and direction of the programme.

Method   To review all the evidence about the operations of the programme in its context.

                              To identify the implications for programme organisers in relation to their current expectations and objectives.

                              To hold discussions with programme organisers about the findings from the evaluation and their significance.

                              To incorporate these findings in a report with recommendations for future policy and action.

---

organisers will rarely be working with a predetermined model of the programme and its organisation. Rather they will be evolving their own model in response to particular local circumstances, opportunities and constraints. This model may or may not be explicitly stated and shared. In any event, it will need testing in the light of how the programme actually operates and is perceived to operate by the organisers, staff and representatives of collaborating agencies. Until this is done, evaluation will lack a firm grounding in organisational realities.

Similar considerations apply to a programme's statement of aim. While most programmes in this field are likely to be working towards some stated objectives, these may be expressed in the form of hoped for, longer-term outcomes, e.g. 'reducing HIV transmission', 'containing HIV spread', etc. In the short run, such longer-term outcomes are not measurable and cannot provide a realistic basis for evaluation, or indeed for programme management. The way a programme is actually working in practice is likely to express a variety of more immediate assumptions and principles about how these longer-term outcomes can best be achieved.

The statement of aim which is of most relevance to systemic programme evaluation will be one which sums up the total process by which a system can achieve its objectives. In the case of the Cambridge AIDS Programme the formulation arrived at was 'to facilitate positive change in social consciousness about HIV infection and AIDS among agencies and communities in Cambridge'.[2] The underlying premise was that if this aim was realised, then desired behaviour change leading to reduced transmission and enhanced care would take place.

This statement of aim in turn linked to, and was informed by, the particular organisational model which the Programme had evolved and was continuing to evolve. This could best be described as a 'network model', in which the Programme could be seen as fostering and developing a network of agencies and organisations in the community, working on their own and together to promote and develop initiatives in response to HIV infection and AIDS. The four core elements were both members of, and a resource to, this network. The role of the director was to give leadership in developing the network through facilitating co-ordination and linking, extending the range of activities and agencies involved, maintaining an information base, mobilising resources and monitoring progress. The underlying strategy was to enable agencies and individuals in the community to understand and work with the challenge which HIV infection and AIDS presented to their own interests and concerns. This strategy was in keeping with a particular philosophy of health promotion which aims to influence the framework of information, beliefs, attitudes and policies against which people make choices and take decisions about their own and the community's health.

Neither the organisational model nor the aim could have been realistically formulated at the outset of the evaluation. In fact, they were an output from a disciplined process of discussion and dialogue with the Programme's sponsors, organisers, staff and collaborators. This process was a necessary prelude to establishing a descriptive base-line for evaluation and had to be agreed and 'owned' by those primarily involved. Without this ownership, evaluation can easily become enmeshed in conflicting interpretations of what is and is not relevant and lose its purchase as a contribution to policy, decision and action.

Stage 2: The choice of indicators

The term 'performance indicators' has been widely canvassed recently to refer to variables which can be used to measure changes resulting from the activities of a programme in relation to specified criteria and standards.[3] In a systemic model, the relevant indicators are those which derive from the description of the programme and its aim, and which provide some qualitative or quantitative measure of outputs. If

2. For a fuller discussion of this statement and its operational specification see Armstrong and Hutton (1989).
3. See, for example, Pye and Kapila (1990), pp. 5–6.

such measures are to be of practical value to the programme organisers, they will also need to be related to process variables – those particular features of the programme which are contributing to performance, whether positively or negatively.

The choice of indicators involves the exercise of judgement, about both what is relevant and what is practicable within the time-scale of evaluation. Evidence about possible indicators will be available from the initial work of system description. Asking questions about what representatives of the programme would consider as measures of performance is one way of identifying and testing the working aim of the programme. In building on and supplementing this evidence it is important that the organisers are again closely involved. Unless the indicators chosen have validity for them, the aim of evaluation is unlikely to be achieved.

In the Cambridge study, the instrument developed as a basis for planning subsequent fieldwork was an evaluation profile or grid which specified the relevant parameters or dimensions of the programme to be investigated. These included the value added by the Programme as a whole to the work of its four core elements, the scope and impact of the Programme's work with a network of other agencies and organisations in the community, and the impact of the Programme on awareness of and attitudes towards HIV infection and AIDS in the community generally. Qualitative or quantitative indicators of outputs relevant to each dimension were then devised, together with the sources and methods for generating the information needed. A more detailed description of this process is given in Pye and Kapila (1990).

In identifying specific indicators, it soon became clear that it was necessary to distinguish between three different types of variable. There were primary outputs such as specific changes brought about through participation or association with the Programme and its work, for example in knowledge, attitudes, agency policies or practice. Consequent on these were secondary outputs, for example how employees or clients of an agency were responding to new, proposed, or actual policies and practices. Identifiable changes in individual behaviour related to drug use, sexual practice, occupational health etc. were considered to be longer-term outcomes. Within the evaluation time-scale, and indeed within the Programme's history to date, evidence relating to these longer-term outcomes was either unlikely to be available or very difficult to interpret. Nevertheless, there is still value in specifying indicators of longer-term outcomes to provide a basis for future research and to help in the planning of what has been termed 'prospective evaluation'.

The technical issues involved in selecting indicators can be illustrated by the following example. It might have been tempting to take as a measure of primary outputs evidence of whether or not particular individuals who had been in contact with the Programme had changed their personal beliefs, attitudes or behaviour. However, given the reference to 'social consciousness' in the statement of aim of the Programme, the critical evidence was rather whether, as representatives of the agency or community, they were now seeing their own and the agency's responsibilities, attitudes and practice in a new way, which informed their decisions and action in their professional, occupational or citizen roles.

Stage 3: Generating information

Table 2 lists, under the method for Stage 3, examples of particular instruments which may be used in carrying out fieldwork. What the appropriate range of instruments is and their priority cannot be pre-determined. It will depend on technical considerations – what is most appropriate given the indicators to be measured, as well as on the practicalities of time, access, interpretability etc. For example, in the Cambridge study, extensive, though not exclusive, use was made of focus group discussions. The decision to do this reflected the evaluators' experience that, where attention is being given to social dimensions of perceptions, attitudes and behaviour, the group setting is both more realistic and more illuminative, since it can highlight differences of perspective and can draw attention to common patterns of response. Moreover, within these groups the ways in which representatives of agencies or of the community worked and contributed to the group itself provided a demonstration as well as a description of the impact the Programme was making.

The use of focus group work, however, raises questions of skill and training. Without experience in this method, other approaches may be needed. No single method, however, will be adequate across the range of qualitative and quantitative indicators. It can also be argued that for any qualitative indicator there will always be value in using more than one approach, as a way of building in some degree of internal control.

An equally significant consideration concerns the need for flexibility. The conventional wisdom of much applied social research tends to emphasise standardisation, for example in the design and use of instruments and in the administration of interview protocols. Correspondingly, there is a tendency to separate data collection and data analysis or interpretation rigorously. Within the framework of this model, such a separation is neither practicable nor desirable. In particular, where qualitative methods are being used, fieldwork will often generate new lines of enquiry which supplement or influence the questions one is asking, or the way one is asking them. Interpretation needs to be more continuous than conventional models allow. For example, it was recognition of the significance of the difference between the Programme's work with people individually and work with them as representatives of their agency or community which led to the formulation of the key questions that informed later participant observation in the Programme's activities.

Stage 4: Working at interpretation

By 'interpretation' is meant a process, based on the available evidence, of questioning, integrating and forming judgements concerning the relation between what is happening in and through the work of the programme and its stated aim. At best, this should move beyond description to explanation – from what to why. No interpretation will be complete, only provisional – something to work with and to test. Its value lies in enabling the programme's organisers and staff to be alert and open to new developments and opportunities. In working at interpretation, relevant questions include:

- What common patterns or trends emerge from the fieldwork?
- Are the findings broadly consistent or are there discrepancies?
- Do the findings validate the description of the programme and its aim or are they contradictory?
- What is the relation between positive and negative findings?
- Can one detect factors in the local environment which shed light on the culture and operations of the programme?

It is not possible to provide realistic guidelines for the process of interpretation, since this must depend on the particular theoretical and conceptual framework the evaluators are using. It may be helpful, however, to offer two examples illustrating the systemic approach used in this instance. The first concerns the relation between the Programme and its context.

An overall finding from fieldwork interviews and discussions was the high level of 'expectancy' associated with the Programme. Those who had contact with it consistently appeared to come away feeling optimistic and better about themselves. A question also asked both of and by the evaluators was, why, given the low prevalence of HIV/AIDS in the district, is this programme apparently so acceptable and successful and why is there such interest in it, actually and potentially?[4]

An initial response suggested that this stemmed from the philosophy

---

4. For evidence relating to this assessment, see Armstrong and Hutton (1989), Chapters 5 and 6.

and working style of the Programme and its staff. Subsequent experience, however, tested in later discussions and interviews, implied that the Programme was also responding to a key feature in its context – the expectancy in Cambridge associated with the presence of large numbers of talented young people destined for leadership in the future, and the increasing importance of the area as a thriving, pioneering and enterprising community – the 'Cambridge phenomenon'.

There was, therefore, an important synergy between the Programme's culture and that of much of the community it served. This hypothesis in turn illuminated other findings, for example the combination of the high degree of energy and initiative being mobilised in agencies' responses to approaches from the Programme, alongside evidence of some tendency to bury or suppress more negative feelings and fears. This in turn was seen to have significant implications for the future leadership of the Programme as it expanded deeper into the community.

The second example related to a significant discrepancy between findings relating to the Programme's work within Cambridge Health Authority as against that of other statutory or voluntary agencies. Work with the health service, particularly in the area of occupational health, aroused more resistance and unfulfilled expectations than was the case elsewhere.[5]

This discrepancy could have been interpreted in terms of competitiveness, rivalry and the natural tension between medical and non-medical personnel. But this would have missed an unresolved ambiguity in the Programme's relation to the Health Authority, which was both the major sponsor and an important potential user or 'client'. Much of the tension between the Programme and the Authority could be seen as an expression of this ambiguity, which led to difficulties in collaborative working. In itself, however, this ambiguity had a positive connotation. By not defining too rigidly the contractual relation between the Programme and the Authority, space was created for experiment and innovation, both organisationally and managerially. Once this was grasped, the difficulties could be reinterpreted in a way which enabled staff to rethink their approach to work with the authority in a more creative way.

Stage 5: The implications for policy

The final stage of the model moves from description and explanation towards policy and action. Evaluation cannot, of course, determine the directions of future development that may be needed. But it can address and help to identify implications arising from the evidence

5. See Armstrong and Hutton (1989), Sections 5.29–5.42.

about what difference the programme is making in its context and what it is that is making that difference.

In considering such implications, the evidence needs to be scrutinised again in terms of its particular bearing on programme management and leadership, organisational structures and their definition, and the pattern of resourcing, including staffing, funding, premises and equipment. Attention here needs to be given to reviewing strategies and priorities, particularly in relation to areas of neglect or omission, public relations and relations with other agencies, and initiatives in the community. There will be opportunities to re-examine methods and styles of work, in particular how they relate to the underlying conception of health promotion and associated values or beliefs and possible areas of innovation and experiment. The evidence may also highlight avenues for further research, including prospective evaluation studies.

The work of this stage is necessarily collaborative and the evidence will rarely be conclusive. Collaboration with the programme organisers and staff in discussing the evidence and its interpretation provides a check on the evaluator's own reading of the material, and a means through which those responsible for policy take back the leadership of the process of evaluation themselves as an ongoing task of management.

Systemic evaluation in context

The systemic model of evaluation described sought to address a specific context in which the need for evaluation was seen to arise. This context is not unique to this particular programme and the model evolved, and has been designed, to be usable elsewhere. Any evaluation is, however, necessarily context-specific. It addresses particular questions, which are being asked in particular circumstances and for particular ends. The model presented here is likely to be especially applicable and relevant where a programme or organisational initiative is breaking new ground, especially in the kind of activities engaged in, the organisational relations involved, the underlying conception of health promotion represented, and the relations between the programme and its users, clients, stakeholders and collaborators. The model is also applicable if there is a readiness to work with qualitative as well as quantitative information, to question assumptions, tolerate uncertainties and be able to work openly with interpretation. Finally, the model is relevant if the organisers and stakeholders are themselves committed to learning and approach evaluation primarily as a tool for learning.

The strengths of this model are that it enables those working for and with the programme to clarify their aims and objectives and to distinguish between what can and cannot be known or assessed in any given time-scale, to distinguish, for example, between 'outputs' and 'outcomes'. Those involved will be enabled to identify and assess the significance of the relation between what is happening in the programme and its context in the community, to be alert to unforeseen links between different activities, and to identify points of growth and assess the relative claims of alternative uses of resources. The model helps bring into focus what may be particularly significant about programme leadership and management. It also provides a basis on which policy and strategies can be realistically reviewed, debated and tested. Finally, it encourages an evaluative stance to the ongoing work of the programme and to identifying needs for further research.

The model does, however, have some weaknesses. There are some questions, for example, which such a model cannot answer: in particular, questions relating to longer-term outcomes. The model is necessarily demanding in terms of programme staff's commitment. It requires a willingness to tolerate uncertainty on the part of both the evaluators and the programme organisers and stakeholders. It does not readily lend itself to quantification and involves issues of interpretation which will always be subject to questioning in the light of evidence which will rarely be incontestable. These 'disadvantages', however, mirror the realities in which such programmes are having to operate. It may not be too far from the mark to suggest that the model has at least the potential to enable programmes to make the most of those realities.

References

Armstrong, D. and Hutton, J. (1989) *Ensuring the Future – Evaluation of the Cambridge AIDS Programme.* London, The Grubb Institute.

Pye, M. and Kapila, M. (1990) Evaluation of AIDS health promotion programmes – concepts and the Cambridge study. *HIV/AIDS & Sexual Health Programme Paper 7.* London, Health Education Authority.

CHAPTER FOUR

Evaluation may Change Your Life but it Won't Solve All Your Problems[1]

Sue Scott

The impetus behind this chapter derives from an involvement in the evaluation of Manchester AIDS in Education Group (MAIEG). This involvement consisted of acting as a consultant to the Group during the planning of the evaluation, helping to write the funding application and then managing the evaluation in the capacity of Director of the Centre for Research into Social Aspects of Health (CRISAH) at the University of Manchester. This chapter is not a detailed discussion of the MAIEG evaluation, and especially not of its 'findings'.[2] The concern is rather to discuss some more general issues pertaining to the evaluation of HIV/AIDS health promotion in general and MAIEG in particular.

The evaluation of HIV/AIDS health promotion is, of course, a relatively new area although there has now been discussion of some of the key issues and problems involved (Aggleton, 1989; Kapila, 1988; Armstrong and Hutton, 1989). What is particular to this type of work, however, is the pressure on both workers and evaluators to 'deliver the goods' in the context of a critical health crisis and the perceived need on the part of state and health agencies to manage this crisis (Weeks, 1989). While there are special issues and circumstances relating to health promotion in this area, some of which will be discussed later, there is a great deal to learn from existing work in the fields of health and educational evaluation (Stenhouse, 1975; Aggleton, 1989), from research in the social sciences, especially sociology (Schutz, 1962; Strauss, 1973), and in particular from feminist sociology (SCARS, 1986; Smith, 1988 and Strauss, *et al* 1983).

---

1. This title comes from a number of suggestions for evaluation T-shirt slogans which were made at the HEA Consultation on the Evaluation of HIV/AIDS Health Promotion (May 1990).

2. The first stage of the evaluation was carried out by Paul Kleiman and the second stage by Polly Radcliffe. The stage one report is available from CRISAH, Department of Sociology, University of Manchester.

This chapter then, is about what evaluation can and should be. The first section discusses some of my own experience of research and evaluation, and the significance of taking a feminist standpoint. It does this in order to illustrate the necessary interrelationship between the context in which an evaluation is produced and the perspectives of those involved in its production. The second section focuses on what seems to be a central debate in evaluation generally, and one which is thrown into sharp relief in the context of evaluating HIV/AIDS health promotion: the relative merits of evaluating processes as against outcomes. This section will also explore the different possible ways of carrying out evaluation and the different sets of interests involved. The third part of this chapter discusses the evaluation of MAIEG as a case study in evaluating HIV/AIDS health promotion. The fourth section concludes with a discussion of the usefulness of sociology and feminism to the development of good evaluation practice in the HIV/ AIDS field.

Lessons from the past

My involvement in evaluation has been somewhat reluctant, and began in 1982. My first experience of evaluation was that of being employed as an action researcher/evaluator on a community health project (Scott, 1986 and 1988). This was in many ways a salutary experience, but one which it may be useful to reflect on in this context. The evaluation of this particular community health project had been insisted on by one of the two funding bodies involved. However, the other funding agency was also the employer of the community work team and insisted that, rather than appointing an outside evaluator, an evaluation post should be created within the existing team.

This situation created a number of problems, since one of the funding agencies had a particular interest in the evaluation, including the way in which community health work was conducted in this specific organisational context, whereas the other had an interest in developing and managing community work, and in gaining more resources for this purpose. I was appointed as a member of a supposedly equal team, but the only member with a brief to carry out evaluation. Needless to say, this was an extremely difficult situation to negotiate as a team member employed to 'monitor and evaluate the work of the team'.

In addition, I came from a rather different professional background and was initially seen by some as an 'academic' with no knowledge of community work and therefore no right to appraise it. Luckily, I did have some previous youth work experience and a background in feminist politics which helped me to integrate with the rest of the team to some extent. Further difficulties arose because the evaluation post was advertised some six months after the project had initially been established. A predetermined set of aims and objectives therefore existed which allowed little scope for negotiation. This is of course often the case when an 'outsider' comes in to carry out an evaluation study but is particularly problematic when, on a day-to-day basis, an evaluator is expected to be *subject* to a particular set of rules of operation.

At interview for the post described above, I made it clear that I was primarily a sociologist with an interest in ethnographic research methods (Burgess, 1982) and also a feminist with particular views about the research process. I did this because I did not want the job if what the sponsors really wanted was measurement of 'improved' health behaviour.[3] I felt strongly at this point that academics should not come into community-based projects on an intermittent basis, take the 'knowledge' away, and write up what could be viewed as the definitive objective version of the project. Instead, it seemed important to apply sociological understandings of process and interaction in specific settings in order to be able to demonstrate the development of the project and the day-to-day realities of doing community health work.

In addition, as a feminist researcher I felt strongly, at that point, that researchers should not 'own' the data, and that reports should be negotiated with and fed back to the participants in the evaluation process (Kleiber and Light, 1978; Mies, 1983). Many researchers, not only feminists, would of course agree with this position, but feminist researchers have raised particular questions about the way in which traditional research both objectifies and renders invisible its subjects, especially women (Roberts, 1981; Graham, 1983). Although it was extremely unlikely that any local authority project would be overtly feminist in its orientation, it did at least appear that 'women's health' was to be the major focus in this case, and as the majority of team members were feminists it seemed an ideal opportunity to carry out action research and evaluation which took the interests and needs of local women seriously, rather than imposing external understandings of their health needs. I had had some involvement in the women's health movement and was interested in the extent to which the feminist critique of biomedical 'health' services could be developed into practice. My commitment then as now was to research as praxis – that is, to research that not only identifies knowledge *about* an issue, but which identifies this knowledge *for* a purpose (Stanley, 1990). However, my views about the position of the researcher in the research process and about the proper focus for the production of feminist knowledge have changed, in part as a result of my involvement in the

3.   Indeed I discovered later that my appointment had been contentious because I was a feminist.

evaluation described above. I now feel that it is important to reflect on the evaluation process, rather than simply learn from the content. As I continue to come across examples of further evaluation programmes which are set up in equally problematic ways, it may be useful to outline the main lessons learned from early work on this community health project:

- evaluation should be built in from the outset and should be part of the legitimate workload of the project
- the involvement of an outside evaluator can offer a very useful perspective and need not be threatening. Outside evaluators do not have to be viewed as objective experts – their input can be enabling, rather than merely static description after the event
- what at the time may be felt to be some kind of 'right on' feminist evaluation may in fact be a lowest common denominator approach which leads to the researcher silencing herself in order to give the other project workers a voice (Scott, 1988; Poland, 1984)
- there are always competing versions of what is going on in a given project, and indeed of what the project is actually about. These should form the basis of the evaluation process
- it is crucial that the evaluation takes account of all levels of the organisation and this may in fact mean that an outside evaluator is essential.

I left the project with the view that I would never be involved with evaluation again, but as distance was gained and confidence regained it became clear that the experience might be put to good use. As a result, I agreed to act as an evaluation consultant first to a women's health project and then to a community arts project before becoming involved with MAIEG. A continued involvement in evaluation has convinced me of the importance of this kind of work, but also of the necessity of being aware of the tensions and contradictions involved in it.

Organisational and ideological frameworks

This section will discuss two levels of evaluation – evaluation with a small e and evaluation with a large E (SCARS, 1986). These will be related to sociological understandings of outcome and process. It will then examine some areas which it is important for evaluation to explore, as well as the role of evaluators, workers in evaluated organisations and the relations between them.

Evaluation with a small e is something which we all do routinely as part of our everyday lives by monitoring our 'performance' and practice against a set of prior expectations. This can and should be done systematically. It is not possible to present a blueprint for doing evaluation, as the precise practices will vary with the setting, but there are some basic monitoring practices which can be identified. The most essential part of everyday evaluation is record-keeping, and a work diary, both for individuals and for the project as a whole, is the basic building block. These documents then become, not the truth enshrined, but the means through which changes, developments, problems and issues can be assessed and explored. For example, if the main aim of a particular project is outreach work with young people, but the work diary reveals that a substantial amount of worker time is spent in the office responding to enquiries from other workers, this can then become the basis for a discussion as to *why* this is occurring. If this process does not occur, the danger is that when an external Evaluation (with a large E) occurs, or time to write the final report comes round, what may have been valid shifts away from the original aims can appear as failures because the means of explanation and justification do not exist. The next level in the evaluation process is to make space and time for appropriate individuals (usually project workers) to meet to discuss the development of the work, reassess aims and objectives and negotiate different views of the project as a whole. The third level is to facilitate the writing-up process and, if necessary, to appoint an adviser to offer support to workers who may be relatively inexperienced in this area. If these practices are carried out as an integral and valued part of the project's work they will have positive results in terms of both worker and project development and can also form the basis of an 'Evaluation' when this occurs.

Good evaluation involves an assessment of the context within which any given project or piece of work is set. It includes critical appraisal of assumptions and expectations, and of the organisational and managerial frameworks. It is not the case that evaluation can only be carried out by neutral, objective outsiders, because such people do not exist. However, as a result of my own experience working with the community health project, which enabled me not only to produce evaluation but to act as an outside evaluation consultant, I feel that external evaluation can have an important part to play. In fact, it is a political necessity to carry out evaluation at both levels whenever possible, since certain areas and issues which bear on the work of a particular project are likely to be relatively inaccessible to project members. It is also difficult to be committed to particular ways of working *and* to critically appraise them at the same time. Grass-roots work, especially in the HIV/AIDS field, is very demanding and requires commitment. There is often the classic situation here of not being able to see the wood for the trees. This is not to say that the wood is a static object which only an outside expert can reveal, but that someone less involved in the day-to-day work might well be able to help workers explore the interrelationships between what they are doing and wider issues in ways which both enrich their work and render 'what goes on' in a particular project more accessible to other interested parties. These two levels of evaluation are equally important and should ideally be undertaken in tandem.

There is no distinction between good research and good evaluation, both involve 'finding out' and seeing things in a new way. Both are also about rendering the everyday world problematic (Smith, 1988), rendering the familiar strange rather than forcing new problems and questions into familiar categories. This is especially important in a new field of work because here we have not yet learned what are the appropriate questions to ask. While evaluation may begin with more specific questions than traditional social science research, it works with the same methodological, theoretical and ethical standards. It is often a major problem for both evaluators and evaluated that evaluation is often mystified and set apart. Training and support should be available to break down this mystique and those with vested interests in claiming that evaluation skills are the property of experts alone should be engaged with critically.

Evaluation with a small e should, in my view, be a legitimate and routine part of the health promotion workload, not something which is tacked on as an afterthought or done in a rush in order to write a rationale for continued funding, and certainly not a substitute for good management or worker support. Evaluation with a large E, on the other hand, is often in practice little more than a one-dimensional description of what went on which leaves the reader, or indeed those who have been evaluated, without the tools to make sense of how the process occurred. This is not good evaluation as it gives little indication of how and why certain aspects were selected and therefore became part of 'what was being evaluated'. A good evaluation should not only render the object of the evaluation intelligible, it should also make the evaluation process and the place of the evaluator(s) in that process explicit (Scott, 1984).

Evaluation should never begin with the funders' questions (e.g. how many people have changed their behaviour?). Instead these questions should be evaluated themselves. If a project has worked to a particular brief, it must, of course, be evaluated in relation to it, but evaluation should also point out the limitations of any given framework or *modus operandi* and possibly even suggest alternatives.

Angst about outcomes

My involvement in the evaluation of health promotion, particularly as it relates to HIV/AIDS, has led me to be increasingly concerned about the pressure to see behaviour change as the only valuable product of this process. There is now ample evidence of the weakness of the relationship between knowledge, beliefs and behaviour (Gatherer *et al*, 1979; Holland *et al*, 1990), and yet behavioural change continues to be seen by many as the goal of health promotion. There is a well-developed critique of this approach (Adams, 1985) but, in the context of the current desire to reduce the incidence of HIV infection, workers are under particular pressure to justify their activities in terms of the specific and positive effects they produce.

If informed and appropriate decisions are to be made about the value of HIV/AIDS health promotion, we must move beyond viewing it simply as a 'good thing' and understand its place within wider public health policy. This means examining work critically. It is, however, crucial to understand the conflicts which emerge in this process. Health promotion theory has emerged primarily from debates within the social sciences, as well as the political and social movements of the 1960s and 1970s. This is evidenced by the shift away from the giving of information to empowerment and community action models of health promotion (Homans and Aggleton, 1988). However, structurally and organisationally, health promotion is permitted (and often begrudged) space within the context of a health service which is dominated by biomedical understandings (Stacey, 1988). This situation often produces tensions between health promotion workers and their management and funding agencies, and frequently evaluation becomes the terrain on which this battle is fought out.

The demand for outcome-focused, goal-oriented evaluation is ideological and is rooted in dominant 'scientific' understandings of the nature of truth and proof. HIV/AIDS has illustrated the ways in which scientific discourse produces more 'facts' in the context of uncertainty. It has also illustrated the demand for 'facts' in order to produce certainty and reassurance in the context of a public health crisis (Weeks, 1989). The notion that what is needed in order to be able to assess effectiveness is quantifiable empirical evidence is so deeply rooted in our culture that it often appears to be simply common sense. Biomedicine has tended to lag behind the other sciences in developing a critique of this positivist tradition and tends to apply it even more rigorously to areas outside of its direct professional ambit (for example health promotion) than to medical practice itself.

HIV/AIDS is a heavily medicalised phenomenon, and this too seems commonsensical, although it can be argued that it should more properly be understood as a complex social issue and not as a disease to be controlled (Weeks, 1989; Holland *et al*, 1990). Lack of certainty about the aetiology and epidemiology of HIV/AIDS raises questions about the value of modern medical science in this context. The insecurity which this situation produces has tended to rebound in the area of health promotion, resulting in pressure to produce results and to bring the crisis under control.

I can perhaps best illustrate this with an example. In many contexts, condom use has come to epitomise safer sex, and to be seen as a major solution to the spread of HIV infection. Numerous public health campaigns and health education and promotion strategies have been developed to encourage condom use. The next stage has been to evaluate the success of this 'education' (DHSS, 1987) by attempting to assess and measure condom-related behaviour, among other things. This procedure is, I would suggest, doomed to failure. The Women Risk and AIDS Project (WRAP) now has questionnaire data from 500 young women which includes information about whether they ever use condoms and many of them say that they do. However, the project also has interview data which makes it clear that past condom use reveals little about future use or about the complexities of negotiating their use (Holland *et al*, 1990). Condom use is intimately linked to meanings and understandings which cannot easily be measured, as well as to the exercise of male power. Outcome measures which record only the number of times condoms are used, but which neglect these more 'hidden' influences, provide only a superficial insight into the effectiveness of HIV/AIDS health promotion.

Even if it were decided that quantitative measures were the most useful form of evaluation, it is highly unlikely that HIV/AIDS health promotion projects will have data at their disposal drawn from random samples of the population. This means that it is not possible to assess the significance of the results obtained. This is not to suggest that nothing can ever be measured or counted, but that we must ensure that quantitative tools are used carefully so as not to invest greater value than they deserve in the results obtained. This raises a problem, given that funding agencies and policy-makers may place health promotion workers under pressure to produce 'results', and everyone wants to be able to produce data which enable 'good' work to be replicated elsewhere. We must therefore move beyond spurious attempts to measure outcomes in ways which lay us open to demands to prove that these were the outcomes of health promotion.[4] Poor measurement is worse than no measurement and, rather than being exact and scientific, a focus on outcomes alone is likely to produce shallow results based on inadequate and superficial analysis.

---

4. Human behaviour is too complex to be explained by any single cause. There is, of course, the possibility of having intervention groups and control groups, but this presents major ethical problems.

It is a mistake to focus on outcomes as separate entities for, unless an understanding is developed of the context in which health promotion takes place and the processes through which this work is carried out, even if seemingly positive outcomes are identified, there may be no means of explaining how they arose or how they can be reproduced. Process is simply not recoverable from a list of outcomes (Stenhouse, 1975). For all that, the polarisation of outcomes and process seems to me to be an unnecessary and artificial construction of the situation. The one should not exclude the other and does not need to, as will be shown.

The whole question of the relationship between HIV/AIDS and health promotion has wide-ranging implications which go beyond whether the effects of the health promotion activity can be measured or not. It is always surprising to find how many people, including those committed to empowerment and community action, see behaviour change as the main goal of their work.[5] This inevitably entails a separation between workers and the 'clients' whose behaviour is to be changed. Given the pressure which many health promotion workers are under, and the enormity of HIV/AIDS as both a threat and a reality, this desire for behaviour change is, of course, understandable but it should not be accepted without question.

Health promotion has roots in a radical approach which is critical of victim-blaming and an over-emphasis on individual responsibility. However, knowledge is power, and as long as we feel we have superior knowledge then we are potentially part of a surveillance apparatus (Foucault, 1973). Self-empowerment and community action models may thereby simply become more subtle tools in the fight to change individual behaviour rather than, or perhaps as well as, being part of a consciousness-raising and politicising process. This can be illustrated by the continuing tendency for some health promoters to place 'clients' in a different category to themselves and to use different criteria to evaluate their behaviour. We need to think carefully about what it means to encourage 'choice' but continue to see certain choices as better than others. We all take risks in our lives, and what is an acceptable risk in a particular context will depend on a range of factors. It is important to place these understandings in the context of a particular ideological framework, the rational choice model which has its roots in liberal individualism (Watney, 1990), but which is often presented as being little more than common sense. It is simply unrealistic to develop a yardstick for behaviour in the context of HIV/AIDS and then use it to assess everyone's progress. We must think about the complexities of our own lives and then think about others

5. Discussion at the HEA Consultation on the Evaluation of HIV/AIDS Health Promotion held at Bristol Polytechnic in May 1990.

in the same complex way. We must learn not to use common-sense categories and labels to tidy up the messiness and variety of everyday life.

The above points have been made in order to move away from the polarised view that it is only funders who want outcome evaluation. It has been my experience that, while being attracted to process evaluation, especially to the extent which it seems less threatening, many workers themselves are keen to 'prove' the effectiveness of their work. This is understandable, especially given factors such as lack of support and the need to seek further funding, but the argument here is that these pressures and tensions should be examined as part of the evaluation process rather than being the strait-jacket into which evaluation is fitted.

The focus on process

It has become increasingly common in the community work field to reject outcome-focused quantitative methods of evaluation. The alternative model which is offered corresponds to the 'qualitative' tradition in the social sciences (Filstead, 1970). This has been labelled *process evaluation* and has come to be seen as more attuned to assessing the complexities of health promotion (Aggleton, 1989), and particularly to evaluating the use of the empowerment and community action approaches. Process evaluation is generally understood as a means of answering *how* as well as *why* questions. How did workers set about their task? How did clients respond? It produces a natural history of a project and attempts to explore different perspectives on the task, including those of management, workers and clients. While this approach has more to offer than 'quantitative' outcome evaluation, it is a mistake simply to substitute process for outcome and still expect the 'truth' to emerge.

There are significant ways in which process evaluation can be developed and made self-critical, and these for the most part have remained unexplored. It is this capacity of evaluation to become self-critical which promises most – politically, organisationally and intellectually. This is the area in which evaluation has most to learn from academic sociology. Evaluation strategies and methods are needed which not only show an understanding of the work in its own terms, but which critically appraise the way in which the work was originally conceived.

Four areas central to good evaluation are particularly relevant in HIV/AIDS health promotion. Sociological literature and analysis can make a useful contribution to the exploration of each of these areas of concern. The first of these is the issue of competing versions of reality, which was a major 'problem' which I faced during my evaluation of the community health project. Although we live in a culture which is publicly committed to scientific truth, in our everyday practice we constantly negotiate between different versions of reality (Cuff, 1980; Wesley, 1987). In this evaluation it became clear that the workers, myself included, had rather differing understandings of what the focus of the work was, what it meant to work in a team and, most importantly, what was going on in the everyday life of the project. This kind of difference is generally understood as a problem, as something which produces conflict, but which is not a legitimate topic for evaluation.

No evaluation can embody the whole truth of a project or piece of work, but a good evaluation should be able to negotiate with different versions of what went/goes on. A good evaluation report should reveal the process of its own production in such a way that the reader can read it actively in order to evaluate the evaluation itself and the place of the evaluator(s) within it. This is an aspect of the research process which has been discussed extensively in the sociological literature (Bell and Newby, 1977; Lee, 1974; Smith, 1978; Stanley and Wise, 1983), but which has not yet entered evaluation discourse to any great extent.

The second area which I will comment on is that of negotiation, which is closely linked with what I have said about 'competing versions'. Much community health work and HIV/AIDS health promotion is likely to be interdisciplinary. This can produce different understandings of the work and it contexts which must then be negotiated within the project team. Workers from different backgrounds, often with different professional orientations, bring with them different 'ideologies' of what the work is about and how it should be done, and this helps establish a 'professionalised locale' (Strauss *et al*, 1973). Strauss and his co-workers argue that it is routine practice for personnel to call upon 'rules of practice' to gain what they want, but they go on to suggest that it is not uncommon for there to be negotiation about what these 'rules' are and for them to be 'stretched, negotiated, argued as well as ignored or applied at convenient moments' (ibid, p. 308). Rules require judgement regarding their applicability to a specific case: for example, how much time should be spent with clients as opposed to working with other workers. Or at what point is so little development work being done that the very existence of a 'rule' about it is called into question. In the context of the psychiatric hospital which they studied, Strauss *et al* suggest that the baseline for negotiation is that the staff should have a shared goal (albeit a rather vague and ambiguous one) 'to return patients to the outside world in better shape', and that this 'goal' is the 'symbolic cement' which holds the organisation together. Members of HIV/AIDS health promotion projects are likely to have equally vague shared goals, such as 'to improve local people's knowledge of HIV/AIDS' or 'to reduce the spread of HIV infection in the local population'. This combination of differing professional ideologies and shared but often ambiguous and/or impossible goals is a rich source of evaluation data.

The third concern is the need to focus on the 'organisation' in all its forms, including different understandings of what constitutes 'the organisation' (Scott, 1988). This entails a focus on how the organisation is produced and reproduced at an everyday level. This level of analysis alone, while it may produce interesting and illuminating data, may well be insufficient in terms of negotiating the future shape of a project, or for the purposes of establishing similar work elsewhere. A thorough evaluation should explore the way in which a given project fits (or fails to fit) into the wider organisational framework. There are three main reasons for this. First, because structures such as health authorities and local authorities play a crucial part in shaping health promotion. Second, because no grass-roots project can develop and continue without organisational and institutional support (Kleiman, 1989). Third, because organisational change may be the most common and effective outcome of HIV/AIDS health promotion. This final point illustrates one way in which it may be unnecessary to separate outcome from process, as it indicates an important sense in which process *is* outcome.

The fourth task which evaluation should undertake is critically to examine the ideological, political and policy basis of the project being evaluated. As has already been noted, it is important to take account of the context and to evaluate work in its own terms, rather than against irrelevant or external criteria. Having done this, however, it is the task of an evaluator to move beyond the given parameters of a piece of work to question the rationale for working in a particular way and attempting to achieve certain goals. This can be threatening as it might be seen as questioning the whole basis of HIV/AIDS health promotion. However, it is not enough to see such work as a good thing *per se* and to accept policy-driven demands for behaviour change. Rather, these demands must be set in their social, historical and political context. Then perhaps it will be possible to ask more useful questions and provide more appropriate services.

Conducting process evaluation

This is an appropriate point at which to consider the position of the evaluator in the research process. Many 'academics' become involved in evaluation as a way of bringing research funds to increasingly 'money-hungry' institutions. Evaluation tends to be seen as practical and therefore easier to do, and easier to obtain funding for, than 'real' research. It is important to acknowledge this and so to recognise that evaluators are not neutral observers, but have agendas of their own, such as the pressure to generate research money and produce publications. This does not mean that they do not also have a genuine interest in the work, but that these issues are central to the production of an evaluation and should therefore be recognised.

Evaluators also need to be reflexive about their own position and to understand the potential power which they have. This does not mean that they should render themselves powerless and write themselves out of the report, rather they should write themselves in. It is crucially important for any outside evaluator to understand the context of the work and the constraints and contradictions which shape any project. An evaluator should, for example, understand what it feels like to work under the pressure of fixed-term contracts and short-term funding. Evaluators should also aim to be flexible in the way that they work and in how they adapt the evaluation strategy to changing circumstances. They should also have legitimate access to all parties involved and to meetings at all levels.

Sometimes evaluators may be in a potentially difficult position if they are employed by the project or its funders, as workers may view them as an extension of management. Even if it is not possible for the evaluation to be funded and organised separately, it is still crucial that legitimate access is negotiated with management and funders, and that these parties accept that they too are part of the evaluation process.

Workers often experience evaluation as a millstone round their necks, either as an enormous threat or as something which will solve all their problems by offering the support and ammunition which they feel is needed to facilitate the work. Different levels of commitment to, and expectations of, evaluation may therefore exist. Evaluation should never be threatening as it should not be about blaming individuals for 'failures'. On the other hand, evaluation should never simply be about making workers feel better since it has to be able to question and problematise. These problems can be avoided if workers have adequate support for their work and do not therefore 'need' evaluation to tell them that everything they have done is wonderful. Workers often feel that all problems have to be tidied out of sight of the evaluation because what can be described as organisational problems, are often translated into personality clashes or individualised in some other way (Scott, 1988). A good evaluation should be able to explicate these 'problems' by setting local knowledge (i.e. workers' perspectives) in a wider organisational and institutional framework (Smith, 1978). Evaluation skills and knowledge can and should be shared. There is no excuse for mystification as it is equally important for evaluators *and* evaluated to learn from successes, mistakes and setbacks.

Lessons for the future[6]

The Manchester AIDS in Education Group (MAIEG) was established in October 1986, by a small number of individuals working in the education/health promotion fields. The aim was to develop a strategy which would enable the 350 educational establishments in Manchester to address positively issues concerning HIV infection and AIDS. The formation of the group was prompted by a request to one of the three Manchester health promotion units to provide some support for educational establishments as required by the document *Children at school and problems related to AIDS* (DES 1986). The first meeting brought together an informal group of interested officers and advisory teachers from the Education Development Service (EDS), the Education Department, Manchester City Council, Manchester AIDSLINE and the three district health promotion units, thus establishing the interdisciplinary style which was to characterise the group from the outset. The main aim of the group was to disseminate information about HIV/AIDS as widely as possible within the educational sector using a 'cascade' approach, which basically involves informing/training a number of people and encouraging them to pass on knowledge and information to others in their workplace. In addition, since September 1987 the work of the Group has included the AIDS in Education Team – a small group of seconded teachers appointed by the Education Department, primarily to develop curriculum materials.

While MAIEG has had no formal status in the organisational hierarchies from which its membership is drawn, it did, at a fairly early stage, develop an advisory role to the Education Department via the HIV/AIDS liaison officer, who was also a founder member of the Group. MAIEG was therefore seemingly in a good position with regard to the development of autonomous working practices and creative responses to the need for HIV/AIDS education across the city.

My involvement in the evaluation of MAIEG came about as a result of organising a one-day conference on social aspects of AIDS. After the event I received a phone call from one of the group members who had not been able to come to the conference but who wanted to meet to discuss AIDS education in Manchester. It transpired during the course of this meeting that the Group, or rather some of its members, were keen to reflect on the work of MAIEG to date, and to think about future directions. Work then began with a subgroup of MAIEG to develop an evaluation strategy and to write funding proposals. What was to be the first stage of the evaluation was funded by the HEA from April to September 1989. The North West Regional Health Authority agreed to match this funding, which enabled a second-stage evaluation.

6. This is the title of the MAIEG evaluation report.

The first stage of the evaluation was set up as a retrospective process evaluation of the Group up to the summer of 1989, and came subsequently to be labelled as a microscopic view of HIV/AIDS health promotion (Pye, 1990). The evaluation fieldwork was carried out via in-depth interviews with Group members and other key individuals as well as via documentary analysis of the Group's records. This produced a detailed account of the differing understandings of the nature of MAIEG and of the processes through which it had developed and changed. While this style of evaluation had been clearly laid down in the evaluation strategy, after the report was complete there was some dissatisfaction with it for a number of reasons.

First, some members felt that the report was overly critical of their work. I would argue that this was not the case, as the focus of the 'criticism' was on institutional and managerial arrangements and not on individuals. This situation, however, illustrates well the need which workers feel for support from evaluation when it is lacking from elsewhere. Second, both MAIEG members and senior local authority officers felt that the evaluation lacked teeth, because it did not set out precisely what the Group had achieved. From some parties, this was a call for measures of behaviour change brought about by the Group's work, which as I have suggested earlier is, in my view, an impossible request. From others, it was a desire to have more clearly set out data on the work which the Group had undertaken.

Third, it was felt that the evaluation said little about the relationship between the Group and the district health authorities. This is certainly the case and can be explained in part by the way in which the Group was closely linked to the Education Department. It is possible that the implications of this situation were only fully revealed after the evaluation had been carried out. However, it is my view that this organisational issue should have been more centrally a topic within the evaluation. Fourth, the evaluation could have explored in greater depth competing perspectives on the processes and events it describes, and this might have enabled people to read the report in a more reflexive way.

A final issue concerns a lack of institutional support for the evaluation which led to its policy recommendations being largely ignored. The evaluation had been negotiated by the Group as an autonomous body, which in many ways it is, but it is nevertheless entirely reliant on institutional support in order to function. In retrospect, it would have been better if the whole hierarchy had been part of an evaluation. That way, it would have been prepared to own it and act upon it. This aspect of an evaluation could be treated differently in future.[7]

7. The fact that I am making criticisms of the evaluation should be viewed positively. I would like to take this opportunity to say that it is overall, a good, interesting and useful piece of work for which many of us are very grateful to Paul Kleiman.

It had always been the intention of the evaluation steering committee to move on to a second stage, funding permitting. The purpose of the second phase was to collect data from those with whom the Group had worked in order to evaluate the cascade approach and to ascertain where further input was needed. This stage has only recently been completed and the full implications have not yet been discussed. What follows is therefore a tentative appraisal of the situation.

We currently have data from many of the schools where MAIEG had carried out training sessions with different groups of workers. Questionnaire responses from these schools indicate whether the school concerned has any policy on HIV/AIDS education, and what, if any, work is being undertaken in this area. This data could be described as indicating the outcomes of the work of MAIEG, but it is my view that, while it is important to indicate the extent of the Group's input, in order to be able to plan future work, another stage is needed. This would entail undertaking case studies of a small number of schools in order to explore the complexities of attempting or 'refusing' to put HIV/AIDS education into practice. This would take the evaluation of MAIEG, through the process of explicating the Group, into a tentative exploration of some of the outcomes of the work and the processes which construct and constrain the contexts in which these outcomes occur. This illustrates clearly the interrelationship between process and outcomes, since here process *is* outcome.

Evaluation and everyday life

In this chapter I have suggested that HIV/AIDS health promotion needs an evaluation framework which is reflexive, and which takes account both of the process of its own production and of the context within which the project, and therefore the evaluation, is set. I have drawn on my own experience to illustrate the kinds of problems which may arise if evaluation is poorly integrated, and have set out both the lessons learned and some of the ways in which a 'qualitative' sociological approach can help in the production of illuminating and useful evaluation. A major problem occurs when evaluation is mystified and separated from everyday life. This is particularly problematic in the evaluation of HIV/AIDS health promotion activities because of the 'medicalisation' of the field, and the consequent ideological pressure to construct what counts as valid knowledge in a very limited way.

Evaluation should not be separated off as a discrete area of expertise, but should be firmly located within the social science research tradition. Some aspects of sociological analysis may be useful in the process of explicating 'what is going on' in HIV/AIDS health promotion. I consider the kind of analysis that has been developed by feminist sociologists such as Smith (1988) to be a particularly useful tool for exploring the multi-faceted realities of HIV/AIDS health promotion. She argues that good 'institutional ethnography' means 'finding a method that does not begin with the categories of the discourse . . . Rather it proposes an inquiry intended to disclose how activities are organised and how they are articulated to the social relations of the larger social and economic process' (Smith, 1988). One of the major criticisms levelled at ethnographic research and process evaluation is that no generalisations can be made. It is possible, however, to move beyond description to analysis if we view the everyday world as problematic, and see the individual case study not as an isolated instance but as a point of entry, as 'the locus of experiencing subject or subjects, into a larger social and economic process' (Smith, 1988). Approaching this task with the benefit of a feminist analysis means looking differently at the world, at interaction and at social structure – with an understanding of power and hierarchy, and of the importance of maintaining people as subjects, rather than the objects of study.

I hope that I have shown that evaluation research, while being challenging and demanding, can also be exciting and rewarding. Good evaluation can and should be able both to address and to reformulate policy questions relating to responses to HIV/AIDS and offer all those involved in a particular project a greater insight into the context and process of their work. It should also be able to link both these levels. Evaluation will never simply solve problems, but by problematising 'what goes on' it can produce new understandings which give people useful knowledge rather than rendering them vulnerable.

Acknowledgements

I should like to thank Richard Freeman for encouraging me to write rather than just talk about evaluation.

References

Adams, L. (1985) Health education: in whose interest? Unpublished MA dissertation, University of London.

Aggleton, P. (1989) Evaluating health education about AIDS. In P. Aggleton, G. Hart and P. Davies (Eds.) *AIDS: Social Representations and Social Practices*. Basingstoke, Falmer Press.

Armstrong, D. and Hutton, J. (1989) *Evaluating AIDS Health Promotion Programmes*, London, The Grubb Institute.

Bell, C. and Newby, H. (1977) *Doing Sociological Research*. London, Allen & Unwin.

Burgess, R.G. (1982) *In the Field*. London, Unwin Hyman.

Cuff, E.C. (1980) *Some Issues in Studying the Problem of Version in Everyday Situations*. Occasional Paper, No. 3, Manchester University Department of Sociology.

DES (1986) *Children at School and Problems Related to AIDS*. London, Department of Education and Science.

DHSS (1987) *AIDS: Monitoring Responses to the Public Education Campaign, February 1986 – February 1987*. London, HMSO.

Filstead, W.G. (1970) *Qualitative Methodology*. New York, Markham.

Foucault, M. (1973) *The Birth of the Clinic: an Archaeology of Medical Perception*. London, Tavistock.

Gatherer, A. *et al.* (1979) *Is Health Education Effective?* London, Health Education Council.

Graham, H. (1983) Do her answers fit his questions?: women and the survey method. In E. Garmarnikow *et al. The Public and the Private*, London, Gales.

Holland, J., Ramazonoglu, C., Scott, S., Sharpe, S. and Thompson, R. (1990) *Don't Die of Ignorance – I Nearly Died of Embarrassment: Condoms in Context*. WRAP Working Paper 2. London, Tufnell Press.

Homans, H. and Aggleton, P. (1988) Health education, HIV infection and AIDS. In P. Aggleton and H. Homans (Eds.) *The Social Aspects of AIDS*. Basingstoke, Falmer.

Kapila, M. (1988) *Evaluation of AIDS Health Promotion*. A background paper prepared for the International Scientific Network on AIDS and Reproductive Health. Stockholm.

Kleiber, N. and Light, L. (1978) *Caring for Ourselves*. University of British Columbia Press.

Kleiman, P. (1989) *Lessons for the Future: An Evaluation Study of the Manchester AIDS in Education Group*. CRISAH Working Paper No. 1, University of Manchester.

Lee, J. (1974) Innocent victims and evil doers. Unpublished paper, University of Manchester.

Mies, M. (1983) Towards a methodology for feminist action research. In G. Bowles and R. Duelli-Klein (1983) (Eds.) *Theories of Women's Studies*. London, Routledge & Kegan Paul.

Poland, F. (1984) Breaking the rules: assessing the assessment of a girls project. In L. Stanley and S. Scott (Eds.) *Studies in Sexual Politics*, 4, University of Manchester.

Pye, M. (1990) Paper presented to the 4th Social Aspects of AIDS Conference. South Bank Polytechnic, London.

Roberts, H. (1981) *Doing Feminist Research*. London, Routledge & Kegan Paul.

SCARS (Social Care and Research Seminar) (1986) Evaluation: a do it yourself approach for feminist projects. In L. Stanley and S. Scott (Eds.) *Studies in Sexual Politics*, 4, University of Manchester.

Schutz, A. (1962) Commonsense and scientific interpretations of human action. In A. Schutz *Collected Papers*, Vol. 1. The Hague, Martinus Nijhoff.

Scott, S. (1984) The personable and the powerful: gender and status in sociological research. In C. Bell, and H. Roberts (Eds.) *Social Researching: Politics, Problems and Practice*. London, Routledge & Kegan Paul.

Scott, S. (1986) Managing women's health. In L. Stanley and S. Scott (Eds.) *Studies in Sexual Politics*, 4, University of Manchester.

Scott, S. (1988) An occupational ethnography of a community health project. Unpublished MA thesis, University of Manchester.

Smith, D.E. (1978) K is mentally ill. *Sociology*, **12i**, 23–53.

Smith, D.E. (1988) *The Everyday World is Problematic*. Milton Keynes, Open University Press.

Stacey, M. (1988) *The Sociology of Health and Healing*. London, Unwin Hyman.

Stanley, L. (1990) (Ed.) *Feminist Praxis*. London, Routledge.

Stanley, L. and Wise, S. (1983) *Breaking Out*. London, Routledge & Kegan Paul.

Stenhouse, L. (1975) *An Introduction to Curriculum Research and Development*. London, Heinemann.

Strauss, A. *et al* (1973) The hospital and its negotiated order. In G. Salaman, K. Thompson and M.A. Speakman (Eds.) *People and Organisations*. London, Longman.

Strauss, A. (1983) *Negotiations*. San Francisco, Jossey Bass.

Watney, S. (1990) Plenary address given at the 4th Social Aspects of AIDS Conference. South Bank Polytechnic, London.

Weeks, J. (1989) AIDS: the intellectual agenda. In P. Aggleton, G. Hart and P. Davies (Eds.) *AIDS: Social Representations and Social Practices*. Lewes, Falmer Press.

Wesley, M. (1987) *The Vacillations of Poppy Carew*. London, Black Swan.

CHAPTER FIVE

Illumination, Collaboration, Facilitation, Negotiation: Evaluating the MESMAC Project

Alan Prout

Effective evaluation must be tailor-made to the activities being examined. This statement, so apparently simple and uncontentious, in practice hides a multitude of difficulties and dilemmas. In this chapter I will describe how the problems of fitting evaluation to a particular HIV/AIDS health promotion project (the HEA-funded project 'Men who have Sex with Men: Action in the Community' (MESMAC)) have been tackled at the design phase. At the time of writing, the Project is still in an early stage and I make no claim that the problems discussed here have been successfully solved. Rather, I will describe the overall approach and how it has been developed in relation to the specific character of the MESMAC Project.[1] In essence this 'tailor-making' has involved a struggle to bring together debates about the theory of evaluation with the practical demands of the Project. Theoretically, evaluation methodology presents a confusing, if not contradictory, mosaic of possibilities, rather than a unified and coherent set of principles; practically, MESMAC has a complex structure and its open-ended objectives are not amenable to traditional evaluation strategies.

The solution advocated here draws mainly from an approach to evaluation usually called the 'illuminative paradigm'. This seeks to shed light on the process by which particular outcomes are brought about. But within this broad framework, the style we shall be adopting, and the style which will be discussed here, stresses the collaboration of all the Project members.[2] It emphasises the role of evaluators as partners within the project and suggests that one of their main activities will be to act as facilitators in an evaluation process that is

---

1. This account is necessarily a selective one and a number of important issues are not discussed at all, e.g. methods of data collection and aspects of fieldwork relations.

2. At the time of writing (June 1990) a full-time evaluation worker, Kate Deverall, has just started work on the Project.

shared by all Project participants. Different participants will have different needs in relation to evaluation and, consequently, methods of working, goals and interpretations have to be negotiated. It is, therefore, in the nature of the evaluation that it will develop and emerge alongside, and as part of, the Project as a whole.

The MESMAC Project

In order to set the evaluation issues in context it is necessary to give a brief description of the project. MESMAC is an HEA-funded initiative which aims to work within a broadly defined community development approach to HIV/AIDS health promotion. It is part of a more general HEA 'Men Who Have Sex With Men Project', which, at present, consists of various mass media campaigns. The stated aims of MESMAC are:

- to establish local community initiatives which will explore felt needs in relation to safer sex and work towards meeting these needs
- to produce a training package to equip a core team of facilitators to develop this work as a general resource for safer sex work in various localities in England.

The project originated from a review of safer sex education workshops for gay and bisexual men, carried out for the HEA (Gordon, 1989). The review applied a theoretical framework constructed by French and Adams (1986) to information about safer sex workshops currently under way, in Britain and internationally. The framework distinguishes between three '. . . phases through which an individual group or organisation may pass as they become, or seek to help others become, more empowered in relation to their health status.' (Gordon, 1989). These phases are in turn related to three models of health education: behavioural change, self-empowerment and collective action. Gordon concluded that, on the basis of the information he was able to gather, the majority of workshops taking place employed experimental methods in pursuit of behavioural change, either in individuals or in communities. There is not space here to rehearse in detail the limitations of behavioural approaches to health education; in any case, these are well known. Silin (1987) summarises these as follows:

The instrumentalist assumption that behaviour can be abstracted, analysed and understood apart from the socio-economic context in which it occurs negates the necessity of addressing questions of social identity and the ethical implication for action. The personal is considered separate from the political . . .

Gordon notes that self-empowerment models might begin to redress some of these problems but concurs with Aggleton (1989) and others (Watney, 1989; Patton, 1985) that unless self-empowerment extends into collective action to change social and political circumstances then it could be self-defeating. It is precisely at this level that, without falsely counterposing themselves to behavioural or self-empowerment strategies, community development approaches aim to make an impact. The San Francisco Stop AIDS Project is cited as an example within this mould, in that it attempts to work towards better health by changing social factors. While there are very real differences between gay politics in San Francisco and the much less visible, powerful and cohesive gay communities in this country, it is suggested that an attempt at a community development-based approach to HIV/AIDS education is worthwhile.

The concept of 'community' is of course highly contested, especially in sociology (Bell and Newby, 1971), although workers in the field are often less naïve about it than some sociologists would seem to appear to believe. A number of dimensions of community-based health promotion have been identified within MESMAC, and it is expected that these will be further explored in the course of the work currently under way. These include:

- the notion that 'community can be defined geographically or by reference to interests
- the emphasis on concerns which are held by many members of a community rather than on individuals and their concerns in isolation
- the importance of seeing problems as interlinked and not isolated and compartmentalised as housing, health, education etc.
- the recognition that there are social, economic and environmental influences on health which are often outside individual control
- an appreciation of the fact that the process of working for changes in health is important in itself
- a commitment to value people whatever their background and to countering prejudice and discrimination.

As a result of this thinking, the (then) AIDS and Professional and Community Development Divisions of the HEA, together with two consultants[3] proposed the project which became known as MESMAC. After a consultation weekend in May 1989, a Policy Advisory Group was set up and four local project sites have subsequently been selected

3. Peter Gordon (Family Planning Association) and Hazel Slavin (South Bank Polytechnic).

and funded.[4] These are: the Newcastle Social Services Department, which hosts a programme for men in both urban and rural areas; the Leicester Black HIV/AIDS Forum, which hosts a project to work with the black population in Leicester; the London-based Terrence Higgins Trust, which hosts a project to work with young gay men; and Leeds AIDS Advice, which hosts a project looking specifically at the needs of men in a large city.

Each project site shares the overall aims of MESMAC but has a different management structure reflecting the host organisation (for example, whether it is in the statutory or voluntary sector), different objectives (over which the local projects have considerable autonomy) and different staffing patterns. The day-to-day co-ordination of the project at a national level is being carried out by a team of three health promotion specialists,[5] who also act as consultants to each of the projects individually. In addition, a forum with representatives from wider HIV/AIDS organisations meets from time to time in a consultative capacity.

Each project has a brief to recruit a group of project workers (known as facilitators), provide training for the development of the necessary skills, and provide support for their work. Using community development methods, facilitators may assess felt needs of local gay communities, work with individuals and groups, enable choice and action on safer sex, put groups in touch with each other to develop models of good practice and assist in the development of individual and group action plans.

The general statement of the ethos of the project is that:

> The MESMAC project will attempt to avoid making assumptions about the needs of men who have sex with men in relation to safer sex . . . Instead [it] will make contact with people in each locality through outreach work and work *with them* to explore what *their needs* are and use a variety of methods, working with individuals and groups, to address these needs. MESMAC is concerned as much with *how* the work is done as with *what* is done. (MESMAC, 1990)

Within these broad guidelines, each project has considerable autonomy to explore and develop its own specific objectives and ways of working. It is expected, and intended, that the project will develop in possibly quite diverse and unexpected ways. The project, in this sense, has a deliberately open-ended character.

---

4. In addition, four other projects are sharing training facilities (including training on evaluation) with MESMAC and, although these sites are not included in the formal evaluation design, it is hoped that material from these projects may be shared.

5. Lee Adams (Sheffield Health Authority), Peter Gordon (Family Planning Association) Hazel Slavin (South Bank Polytechnic).

Theoretical and political issues in evaluation

Evaluation was considered essential to MESMAC from the start, but finding a format appropriate to the needs of the project has meant confronting some of the underlying political issues of methodology. While evaluation has recently moved further up the agenda of HIV/ AIDS work, in both the statutory and voluntary sectors, this process has not been without resistance, suspicion or, at the very least, ambiguity. Broadly speaking, the further up the (formal or informal) hierarchies of organisations that one goes, the greater is the enthusiasm for evaluation. Conversely, among grass-roots workers, anxiety about evaluation is often at its highest, centring on the possibilities of surveillance and control which it is often taken to imply. Such responses are entirely understandable, given the dominant purposes and ethos of evaluation research. These have recently been scathingly characterised by a sociological critic (Prior, 1989) as part of the rationalisation and commodification of human attributes and activities in modern societies.

Mainstream evaluation methodology (see, for example, Rossi *et al*, 1979) claims to be a scientific method for the objective, neutral and rational assessment of human performance; its focus is on the efficient and effective achievement of preordinate objectives, typically defined as the only appropriate outcomes of work, and the main interest of evaluators is their accurate measurement. Many in education, health care and social work resent the reduction of the complex, multi-faceted and emergent human activities that constitute their work to items such as 'performance indicators' and 'input and output measures'. Prior's critique resonates with these feelings, and suggests that evaluation techniques are not much more than an ideological mask for managerial control and the interests of the powerful.

As a critique of *mainstream* evaluation research, his account is a persuasive one. What, however, it fails adequately to recognise is the extent to which evaluation researchers (especially in the field of education) have already made a powerful critique, and have developed alternatives to it. These alternatives cannot claim to have resolved the many dilemmas which evaluation poses, but they do at least engage with dominant approaches, contesting the terrain it seeks to monopolise.[6] They do so by suggesting methods of evaluation, which are more subtle (and therefore more adequate to complex fields of

---

6. The illuminative paradigm has had a profound effect on educational evaluation. Political trends in the 1980s, however, have created a tension between the values of 'the alternative tradition of evaluation . . . and the requirements of those currently funding the majority of evaluation activity in the UK' (Hopkins, 1989). Hopkins offers a practice of evaluation for development which attempts to grapple with these tensions and in this sense is rather similar to the position advocated here.

activity such as health care and education), and more open to the many different viewpoints and interests that are represented there. Their promise is to allow other perspectives, especially those of grass-roots workers, to have a voice in evaluation. They pay far more attention to contextual and 'political' factors, such as the adequacy of resources, pressures from competing demands on workers' time, and needs around professional development. Their general strategy is to examine processes (how and why work is done) as well as the outcomes of particular initiatives.

In the health services these alternatives have not found much expression (but see Smith and Cantley, 1985). However, in social work (Lishman, 1984) and, most markedly, in education, oppositional approaches have a considerable history and tradition. In fact it was in education that the first critiques of the dominant paradigm were made (see, for example, Stenhouse, 1975). Much of the material that came from the first wave of critical discussion was brought together in a collection entitled *Beyond the Numbers Game* (Hamilton *et al*, 1977). The editors of this volume argue against what they call the 'agro-botanical' approach to evaluation (which is roughly speaking similar to the dominant tradition criticised by Prior) and call for a shift to 'illuminative' evaluation. This, they argue, should be concerned with description and interpretation, rather than measurement and prediction. It should deal with the processes within a learning milieu (how and why things happened in a particular way) and attempt to illuminate the complex array of questions that arise in such processes, as well as the multiple outcomes which may emerge. It should recognise that within such settings there are many often competing interpretations, depending on different actors' points of view. Evaluation should acknowledge this rather than claiming objective insight.

In the remainder of this chapter I will outline the approach to evaluation that is being taken within the MESMAC Project and discuss the process by which it was arrived at. I want, however, to place this approach within the wider issues which I have raised above, suggesting that it is possible to practise a form of evaluation which, while recognising managerialist concerns (as well as wider ones of public accountability), places these alongside other interests, such as those of grass-roots workers, allowing each to speak through the process of evaluation. Such an approach must of necessity be reflexive; that is to say, it must self-consciously place evaluation within (rather than outside) the programme it is evaluating and remain aware that it is part of, not apart from, the personal, political and professional processes of the project.[7]

---

7. The personal, political and professional are, of course, interlinked.

Evaluating MESMAC

HIV/AIDS health promotion raises issues around the politics of sexual orientation, gender, class and race. The field is subject to shifting and profoundly ambiguous social and cultural attitudes. As a community development project, MESMAC addresses itself directly to these issues and as such might be seen as especially vulnerable to attack. The work is, therefore, difficult and sensitive. In these circumstances evaluation must be aware of the potential it has for adding to or reducing these difficulties. Both the role of evaluation in the representation of the project and the impact of evaluation on the internal relationships of the project should be considered when deciding its form and content.

The first issue which followed from the political context of the Project was the overall style of the evaluation. The stance of the dominant paradigm, as discussed above, is that of 'neutral observer', rationally judging the success of the project in effectively and efficiently achieving its stated objectives. In some ways this is a tempting position to claim. In terms of the public presentation of a project, for example, evaluators can claim distance and this is often seen as having political utility, especially when allied to notions of academic disinterest and scientific measurement. Internally to the project, however, the effect of this stance can be to short-circuit debate about the project and its conduct by imposing an 'authoritative' view.

But while this position appears to carry some (at least short-term) benefits within the political context of AIDS/HIV work, it also has enormous problems. At the most general level it is a style of work which tends to reinforce what has recently been called 'disciplinary', as opposed to community-based, health education (Watney, 1989), and, as such, it contradicts the ethos of the MESMAC Project. In theoretical terms it ignores debates in the evaluation (and broader social scientific) literature which question the very notion of an objective observer. In practical terms the adoption of such a mask within the Project would also have effects on the relationship between the evaluator and the evaluated (and in this sense the claim to neutrality is bogus indeed). The aim of MESMAC is to provide a framework within which the HIV/AIDS needs of gay and bisexual men can be explored and met in dynamic and creative ways. The 'neutral' evaluator, who has no involvement in the development of such work, who is tied to relatively static notions of what should be achieved within the project, but who simultaneously holds a powerful position of judgement, would be in serious danger of distorting and inhibiting what the Project is setting out to do.

These considerations suggested that the evaluation could not have a neutral relationship to the Project. The question therefore arose as to how a more constructive role might be entered into. One way of thinking about this was to use the distinction between formative and summative evaluation. In the former mode, part of the evaluator's role is to give feedback at all stages and levels of the project, supplying a continual stream of constructive criticism throughout the project. In the latter, the emphasis is on making overall judgements at the end. The formative role, however, places the evaluator clearly *within* the project rather than as an commentator on the outside. It also raises issues about what sort of feedback should be given.

Because of these issues, MESMAC seemed better suited to an illuminative style of evaluation, and this contention was reinforced by considering another feature of the Project: its concern to identify 'good practice'. This is a problematic notion in itself, and one to which I will return. At this point I want to emphasise that identifying 'good practice' involves documenting the project in a comprehensive way. As a minimum, both *process* and *outcome* should be examined. The most telling weakness of outcome-only evaluation is that it assesses without explaining and therefore only very limited lessons can be drawn from it (Stenhouse, 1975; Hamilton *et al*, 1977). In the case of MESMAC a description of processes was thought vital. The diffusion and application of examples of 'good practice' rely on a knowledge of the 'how' and 'why' of practice: why the project was conducted the way it was, what obstacles were met and how they were overcome, what resources are needed for success, etc. All these questions concern process rather than outcome.

Similarly, when it came to outcomes the illuminative style seemed more appropriate to MESMAC. As a project it is concerned with two main types of outcome. On the one hand, some predetermined or *preordinate* objectives are required, if only as one of the grounds on which systematically to compare local projects. On the other hand, a *responsive* evaluation needed to leave room for outcomes which were unplanned and emergent, or simply specific to the diverse local projects. Whatever design was to be adopted would have to be capable of attending to both types of outcome.

A final difficulty, alluded to above, was that MESMAC involves several interlocking levels of activity. This demanded that several, distinct but not separate, evaluations be carried out simultaneously. The local projects are diverse in character, and require a mixture of evaluation criteria and methods, some responsive to the particular local situation and others preordinate to it. The levels involved are:

- the national strategic level, focusing mainly on the Project Advisory Group and its actions
- the level of local initiatives and their conduct
- the level of comparative analysis between the local initiatives.

Combining these levels into a coherent whole was clearly going to be a complex task, one perhaps too large for an evaluator working alone to encompass. If this was to be so, then it once again raised questions about the relationship between the evaluator and other project participants; specifically it suggests the need to see evaluation as a collaborative task.

Collaboration, negotiation and facilitation

MESMAC is a multi-level, diverse and complex project. The task of evaluating was going to involve working within a number of tensions, between:

- the demand for an outside view and the need for sympathetic engagement in a difficult piece of work
- formative and summative tasks
- process and outcome
- preordinate and responsive outcome dimensions
- the different levels of the project and their diverse needs

This last section lays out some of the ways in which, by stressing the role of collaboration, negotiation and facilitation, the evaluators are currently attempting to work within these tensions.

The first and most important principle that has emerged so far is that the work of the formal evaluation will be integrated with evaluation activities carried out by the local project facilitators themselves. Evaluation will, given the exploratory character of the Project, be a central and continuous part of the work of local facilitators. Project development is a reflexive not a mechanical task, requiring participants to go through a continual cycle of planning, action and reflection (Stenhouse, 1975). It would be a pointless duplication of effort for this to take place in isolation from the formal evaluation. A good illustration of the potential for collaboration between the evaluator and the local projects can be gauged from the work of the Sheffield AIDS Education Project, an example from which MESMAC (and others) can learn. The project workers there carried out self-evaluation based on imaginative, sensitive but rigorous record-keeping. They have been able to build up an extremely rich and flexible resource from which to draw when evaluation is needed. Not only have they recorded (in ways which assure the anonymity and confidentiality of clients) the number and types of client with whom they worked and the outcomes of that work, they have also tracked the context and processes involved, including their own feelings and responses to their work.[8]

The quality of both the evaluation and the local projects may be enhanced by working in a collaborative way. It provides an opportunity for both self-evaluation and the 'quick and dirty' feedback which the evaluation literature (MacDonald and Walker, 1976; Fullan, 1982) suggests is essential for useful formative evaluation. It would, however, be self-deceiving to see only benefits in collaboration. The evaluator is in effect trading off the mask of neutrality for a closer relationship with the project participants. This may entail living with and juggling tensions and divided loyalties.

If collaboration is to take place, then a priority task for the evaluation is the negotiation of guidelines on the respective roles, duties, obligations and working practices of the evaluator and other project participants. Such agreements cannot be laid down in advance but must be negotiated according to the wishes and preferences of the parties concerned. It is clear, however, that a process for this negotiation must be established as a routine part of the evaluation. Experience of this so far suggests that the negotiation of boundaries is central to this process – boundaries around confidentiality, gaining permission to collect data, and securing the release of information and interpretation. Such negotiated boundaries are essential to developing trust and respect, but they too may involve trade-offs. Some aspects of the project, for example, may be negotiated out of the documentation. Clearly there must be limits to this, although they are hard to specify in advance. Adherents to conventional evaluation may be shocked by such a suggestion but in reality they are in a similar position. They too close off topics for inclusion by the adoption of a distanced stance from project participants, who may be unwilling to discuss aspects of their work.

Collaboration would also seem (at least in the case of MESMAC) to imply a facilitation role for evaluators. If the project workers are to become reflective and self-evaluative, then the evaluators may (where appropriate) need to become involved in training in evaluation concepts and techniques. At the very least, evaluators will have to be involved in discussions about how records are kept by the project workers and managers and how these will relate to the formal evaluation. At its most productive, this could become a task of sharing the detailed design of evaluation. This would be a two-way exchange: project workers would be empowered to place their concerns on the evaluation agenda and to engage in the evaluation of their own work, as well as the conduct of the overall project; evaluators would have

8. I am grateful to Jef Jones, Greg Foister and Jo Adams for sharing their working methods at an evaluation training workshop for AIDS/HIV workers held in April 1990.

much to learn through this process which would enrich evaluation data. One consequence of a facilitative style, however, is that evaluators have to be ready to accept that their own actions too may become the focus of evaluation.

Negotiation and facilitation are also important when it comes to identifying 'good practice'. The definition of 'good practice' is problematic and may be judged quite differently by different participants in the project. Why, from among all the plurality of viewpoints within the project, should an evaluator be accorded uniquely prescient insight? A more realistic aim might be to record and provide a commentary on the different interpretations of good practice that arise, feed them back for more general discussion and report the outcome of this process. It is far from clear that such a discussion will lead to consensus, but the clarification of positions and viewpoints will contribute to understanding the dynamics of the project.[9]

This way of working might also be made to coincide with another aim of the evaluation: to provide a comprehensive account of the work of the project. Indeed, identifying good practice seems to imply the need for a comprehensive account since it requires a good deal of contextual material: the conditions under which the project took place, the practices adopted by the project participants, and their relationship to its stated objectives of the project(s), as well as its emergent or unintended outcome. A range of alternative 'process' models, all associated with an illuminative approach to evaluation (Stenhouse 1975; Hamilton *et al*, 1976; McCormick 1982) is available. In work evaluating MESMAC, the decision was taken to adopt the model put forward by Stake in 1967. While not beyond criticism, Stake's framework is something of a classic of the illuminative tradition. It is especially salient to MESMAC because it provides a comprehensive framework, within which outcomes and processes can be contained.

Stake achieves comprehensiveness by introducing two sets of distinctions which together make up his concept of a 'description matrix' of any educational initiative. The first distinction is between the *intended* and the *observed* practices: that is, the difference between what is planned to take place and what actually happens when those plans are put into practice. The second set of distinctions is that between three aspects of the process: antecedents, transactions and outcomes. Stake (1967), writing about educational contexts, defines these terms as follows: *antecedents* refer to 'any condition existing prior to teaching and learning which may relate to outcomes'; *transactions* refer to 'the countless encounters of students with teacher,

---

9.   There are a number of complex methodological points implied here and I do not mean to indicate that there is a unitary truth about the project. Accounts will depend upon who is saying what to whom and under what circumstances. See, for example, Hammersley and Atkinson (1983).

student with student, author with reader, parent with counsellor – the succession of engagements which comprise the process of education'; and *outcomes* should be interpreted in the widest sense, including outcomes which are 'immediate and long-range, cognitive and conative, personal and community-wide'.

Clearly these terms require a good deal of adaption to the context of a community development process but, granting that this is possible, then putting these two sets of distinctions together gives the content of what Stake calls a 'description matrix' (Figure 8).

Figure 8 **Description matrix in Stake's evaluation model**

Intended antecedents $\longrightarrow$ Observed antecedents

Intended transactions $\longrightarrow$ Observed transactions

Intended outcomes $\longrightarrow$ Observed outcomes

By expanding the range of data collected in this manner, the evaluation will be able to provide insights into process which may be important to the definition(s) of good practice. The processes and practices of the project can be interrogated by asking questions about:

- the aims and strategy of the project, their coherence and realism, the factors that shaped their formulation either as constraints or enablers
- the factors that in practice facilitated and inhibited the achievement of the aims and the way in which the strategy worked
- the kinds of new experience and understanding that were gained in the process of putting the strategy into practice
- the broader lessons for community-based HIV/AIDS education that can be learned from the project.

Each of these questions can be addressed to every level of the project: participants and facilitators in local projects, host organisations, the advisory group, the forum members, HEA officers etc. It is to be assumed that different perspectives will be generated by different actors in the project and that these will lead to different judgements about overall success or failure. In this sense no 'objective' criteria for good practice can be established.

The 'viewpoint matrix' that these different perspectives suggest can then be used to illuminate the different definitions of good practice that the Project is likely to generate.

Stake's model is also helpful in suggesting a way of dealing with the complex issue of outcomes. The aims and objectives of the Project, described earlier in this chapter, form the intended outcomes of the project. As such, they comprise an initial set of definitions against which preordinate evaluation criteria (one type of outcome) can be generated for purposes of comparison between projects. Each local initiative could be looked at in terms derived from these: numbers of people involved in educational/training activities; the effectiveness of the activities gauged according to self-reported changes in knowledge, agency referral, understanding, empathy, skill, and actual and intended changes in conduct; and the efficiency of initiatives gauged by the ratio of resources to effects.

Indicators such as these would be at the centre of an evaluation carried out within the dominant paradigm, and they also have a place within the approach we are taking to the evaluation of MESMAC. However, other, perhaps more important, outcomes cannot be dealt with in numerical terms. Data will also be collected on such factors as: the degree of engagement with other community organisations; the development of new understanding about the needs of men who have sex with men in relation to HIV/AIDS and safer sex education; the development of innovative strategies for group and individual action on HIV/AIDS and safer sex practices; the durability of initiatives and their prospects for longer-term work; the impact of initiatives on the local political environment in which HIV/AIDS education takes place; and the practice of equal opportunities.

Stake's model, with its distinction between intended and actual outcomes, however, strikes a note of caution in relation to any attempt to specify too closely any list of possible outcomes. There may be many other, as yet unforeseen outcomes, to the Project. Indeed, to some extent it would be disappointing if there were not, given the exploratory and innovative aims of the MESMAC Project. A key task of the evaluation will, therefore, entail being sensitive to, and documenting, the emergence of these outcomes. Stake's concepts are helpful in this task since they keep emergent outcomes permanently on the evaluation agenda.

Finally it is intended that the evaluators take on the same facilitation role over outcomes as was proposed in relation to process. In part this will involve collaborating with project workers in relation to records and documentation. It will also consist of facilitating project-wide discussion on the outcomes of MESMAC as a whole. This may appear relatively straightforward, but in practice it is likely that here too differences in interpretation will arise. Even apparently simple numerical measures are subject to this. For example, from the list given earlier, what duration and type of client contact should count as being 'involved in educational/training activities'? Any interpretation offered should be treated as a basis for further discussion rather than a definitive statement.

Conclusions

The MESMAC Project presents a unique combination of problems for evaluation. This chapter has explored how one attempt to meet these problems has been arrived at. Its starting point, and main inspiration, is the illuminative paradigm, and in this sense it imports into the HIV/AIDS field a tradition which originated within education rather than the health service. However, certain aspects of the illuminative approach have been modified or emphasised in order to fit the particular needs of participants in the MESMAC Project. First, a concern with process has not been allowed to exclude the importance of outcomes. Second, those features of the illuminative paradigm which stress the role of evaluation in project development have been emphasised. As a result, evaluation is seen as having a definite (though far from exclusive) role in facilitating, negotiating and collaborating in the work of the Project. This is very different from traditional notions of external evaluation and, although it will no doubt raise a multitude of difficulties and dilemmas, it also promises a more productive relationship to the work that is being undertaken and the drawing of lessons from it.

References

Aggleton, P. (1989) Evaluating health education about AIDS. In P.J. Aggleton, G. Hart and P. Davies (Eds.) *AIDS: Social Representations, Social Practices*. Basingstoke, Falmer Press.

Bell, C. and Newby, H. (1971) *Community Studies*. London, Allen and Unwin.

French, J. and Adams, L. (1986) From analyis to synthesis. *Health Education Journal*, 45, 2, 71–4.

Fullan, M. (1982) *The Meaning of Educational Change*. New York, Teachers College Press.

Gordon, P. (1989) Safer Sex Education Workshops for Gay and Bisexual Men: A Review. London, Health Education Authority, mimeo.

Hamilton, D. *et al* (Eds.) (1977) *Beyond the Numbers Game: A Reader in Educational Evaluation*. Basingstoke, Macmillan.

Hammersley, M. and Atkinson, P. (1983) *Ethnography: Principles in Practice*. London, Tavistock.

Hopkins, D. (1989) *Evaluation for School Development*. Milton Keynes, Open University Press.

Lishman, J. (Ed.) (1984) *Evaluation Research Highlights in Social Work*, 8. London, Jessica Kingsley.

McCormick, R. (Eds.) (1982) *Calling Education to Account*. London, Heinemann Education.

MacDonald, B. and Walker, R. (1976) *Changing the Curriculum*. London, Open Books.

MESMAC (1990) *First Report*. London, Health Education Authority, mimeo.

Patton, C. (1985) *Sex and Germs: The Politics of AIDS*. Boston, South End Press.

Prior, L. (1989) Evaluation research and quality assurance. In J.F. Gubrium and D. Silverman (Eds.) *The Politics of Field Research: Sociology Beyond Enlightenment*. London, Sage.

Rossi, P.H. *et al* (1979) *Evaluation: A Systematic Account*. Beverly Hills, Sage.

Silin, J. (1987) The Language of AIDS: public fears, pedagogical responsibilities. *Teacher's College Record*, 89, 1.

Smith, G. and Cantley, C. (1985) *Assessing Health Care*. Milton Keynes, Open University Press.

Stake, R.E. (1967) The countenance of educational evaluation. *Teacher's College Record*, 68, 523–44.

Stenhouse, L. (1975) *An Introduction to Curriculum Research and Development*. London, Heinemann.

Watney, S. (1989) Taking liberties: an introduction. In E. Carter and S. Watney (Eds.) *Taking Liberties: AIDS and Cultural Politics*. London, Serpent's Tail.

CHAPTER SIX

Evaluation not Reaction –
The Evaluation of Local Authority
HIV/AIDS Training and Health
Education Programmes

Wendy Clark

There are three reasons why HIV/AIDS training and health education in local authorities is highly important. First, local authorities are major providers of services. Second, they are major employers in particular geographical areas and, finally, within those areas, they are key opinion leaders with the potential for considerable influence in the local communities they serve. For these reasons, the various HIV/AIDS training and health education initiatives that many local authorities have been involved with deserve particularly close scrutiny.

At the end of 1989, the HEA in conjunction with the Local Government Training Board (LGTB) produced a publication for local authority staff who were involved with, or intending to develop, HIV/AIDS training and health education programmes. Entitled *HIV Infection and AIDS: A Training Handbook for Local Authorities*, this document examines the component part of an HIV/AIDS training process and its findings are intended to assist local authorities to look closely at what they have been doing and to plan for the future (Clark, 1989).

All the training programmes examined in this publication work from the assumption that staff education and training on issues to do with HIV/AIDS result in increased knowledge, enhanced awareness and understanding, and a better quality service for clients. One of the major aims of the research that underpinned the development of this publication, and with which I was associated, was to examine the kind of training already under way, with a view to identifying which kinds of training achieved their goals and which kinds did not. While this chapter will identify the main findings in the publication, it is important to point out that the purpose for which the handbook was developed meant that the research leading up to it involved little by way of systematic quantitative data. A major objective was to produce a 'user friendly' resource that could be used easily by local authority

staff and other organisations in order to help them set up training and
plan for the future. Hence the analysis offered here will be largely
qualitative and will describe some of the main techniques used to
evaluate training, as well as the options that need to be explored more
fully in the future in order to ensure that training does what it is
intended to do.

Training responses

The main findings from the survey of local authority provision
suggest that the majority of local authorities in England and Wales
have so far done relatively little to respond to HIV/AIDS, either in
their service provision or by providing staff training and education.
Additional evidence for this was provided by the discussions that
took place as part of the regional dissemination events associated
with the launch of the publication in 1989/90. Constant press
misreporting on HIV/AIDS, coupled with a general weariness with
the subject and the substantial changes in local government, have
meant that HIV/AIDS training has slipped even further down the
majority of local authorities' agendas. Those few authorities that
have done a great deal of HIV/AIDS training mostly undertook the
work between 1986 and 1988, coinciding with the period immediately
after the government's first public information campaigns. Whether or
not training has been undertaken is closely related both to the local
prevalence of HIV/AIDS and to management perceptions of the present
and future significance of the epidemic. Additionally, pressure from
local voluntary groups, the dedication and perseverance of individual
officers or counsellors and the degree of 'crisis' experienced by the
authority have all acted as contributory factors in prompting local
training responses.

The quality of training offered has been substantially influenced by
co-operation between different bodies and within local authorities
themselves. At an individual level, and in authorities that have
mounted HIV/AIDS education and training programmes, contacts and
co-operation have generally been good, but at an organisational level
there have been substantial boundary conflicts. Training quality has
also been influenced by the background and experience of those who
have run programmes. All too often those facilitating training events
have been local authority HIV/AIDS advisers who may or may not
have prior training experience, or people with limited expertise in HIV/
AIDS, others who have 'done an HIV/AIDS course or two' or people
drawn from the voluntary sector. Generally, those involved have not
been experienced trainers themselves, and relatively few central
training sections or mainstream trainers in local authorities have so far
been involved in work of this kind. On the whole, HIV/AIDS training

tends to be seen as 'low status', 'too specialist' or 'boringly repetitive'. As a result, it tends to be marginalised and cut off from other training activities. There is also something of a tendency for HIV/AIDS trainers to lack status and credibility within local authorities. Where they have status, it is related to the degree of management support they receive and the interest shown by those in senior positions.

Additionally, within some local authorities a growing number of training programmes are facilitated by outside organisations. Here, quality control may be poor and the kind of training participants receive may vary considerably depending on the approach of the trainer. Trainers themselves report that their work is extremely stressful and does not receive adequate support. Occasionally this can be because the trainer is unable to distance him or herself from a subject in which there is too strong a personal investment, although often it is related to the fact that local authorities underestimate the kind of consultancy, supervision and support that is needed in relation to work of this kind. All those involved in local authority training programmes report a consistent lack of commitment and involvement by management at all levels.

Because much HIV/AIDS training has arisen as a response to a crisis, rather than in a more considered way, many programmes have been set up without a training needs analysis having been carried out beforehand. Few HIV/AIDS trainers have had the necessary organisational and political understanding and skills to be able to argue for time to do this before starting training itself. It is also true that, because of their relative inexperience, job history etc., relatively few HIV/AIDS trainers, advisers, co-ordinators and workers have prior experience in training needs analysis, evaluation or training audit work. Such problems tend to be compounded by the fact that many of the individuals concerned are offered little by way of induction that would allow them to learn the complexities of local authority webs and networks. As a result, HIV/AIDS training is often provided in an undifferentiated way with all employees receiving similar input, regardless of their needs.

Much HIV/AIDS training invites little active participation from learners, with directed courses ranging in length from a few hours to several days. There is not much indication of a more radical approach being used and new training initiatives seem not to have influenced that which is provided. There is also something of a tendency for HIV/AIDS training not to be as job-related as many other courses. It also makes particular demands on participants, who may be unfamiliar with work around health education, attitude awareness and anti-discrimination. Without adequate advance preparation, difficult issues can arise. Additionally, work on HIV/AIDS often takes place in the context of public perceptions and media responses which make it hard for participants to be rational. Ultimately work of this kind needs to be normalised into the organisations in which it takes place and not sensationalised. There are, however, some extremely positive off-shoots arising from HIV/AIDS training in local authorities. In particular, some courses hold the potential to challenge accepted practices and attitudes towards the services and training that local authorities provide.

Finally, there is little evidence that local authority HIV/AIDS training is being evaluated in any systematic way. Any evaluation that is taking place is generally limited in scope to the training event itself and fails to recognise that an event is part of a wider process, not an end in itself. Only rarely are there policies or local authority statements to underline and reinforce key issues that arise in the training context (cf. Jackson, 1988).

Existing approaches to evaluation

Over the years there has been a considerable amount of training in local authorities – more than enough to be able to carry out the kinds of evaluation and training audits that are needed in order to learn what is needed in the future. As yet, however, little of this information is available, since few local authorities have a culture that values the evaluation of training or services, be this internal or external. But the culture is beginning to change, and increasingly the move is towards quality assurance, performance indicators and the implementation of new evaluation techniques. The danger is that, because HIV/AIDS trainers tend not to be linked into broader training functions, they may fail to engage with these new priorities.

Training evaluation, if it is carried out at all, is mostly confined to asking 'How enjoyable was the course?' This satisfaction factor is usually evaluated in a highly subjective way by asking participants to respond to a number of relatively closed questions. Little attempt is made to separate an evaluation of the training course from the process of training itself; what is looked at and commented on by participants is just one part of a complex interrelated system. This kind of evaluation generally produces responses of the kind that indicates that the training was 'OK', that it was 'liked' or that it was 'enjoyed'. It does not measure the extent to which the organisation's needs have been met or validated, as successful outcomes are presumed to reside entirely in the positive comments emanating from the glow of post-course satisfaction. When negative comments are made, they tend to take the form of complaints about the environment and about what has been left out of the training – safe areas which destroy neither the trainer's confidence nor the group euphoria that may exist at the end of a course.

Many of the groups currently being trained in local authorities are staff such as manual workers who, prior to HIV/AIDS training, have had few other training experiences. Because of this, work around HIV/AIDS can often be seen as a threat, since participants have little to compare it with. As a result of training, many of these fears and anxieties may be allayed by feelings of having been comfortable, of not having been exposed and of not having had to 'learn' anything. Much of this ignores the fact that good HIV/AIDS training should respond to organisational needs not just individual anxieties, and it is these organisational needs that are so rarely examined by existing systems of evaluation.

Matters are further complicated when organisations fail to specify their objectives clearly in the first place. Sometimes this lack of clarity may be the responsibility of those doing the training, even if they are working in relative isolation from other parts of the authority. But in these circumstances it is all the more appropriate to set specific targets and objectives. Part of the problem here relates back to the fact that many local authority HIV/AIDS advisers are not 'trainers'. They may lack the skills necessary for strategic planning and the development of innovative training programmes. HIV/AIDS training, too, is rarely given enough resources to allow adequate consultation and preparation beforehand. However, training and education in local authorities should be a serious business, since its costs are considerable – both financially and in terms of human resources and service delivery. Leaving things to chance or to natural processes is unprofessional and can border on negligence.

Barriers to better practice

A range of issues needs to be addressed by local authorities if they are to successfully evaluate the HIV/AIDS training they provide. One of the major barriers to the development of systematic and strategic approaches is the trainers' view of training. Many HIV/AIDS trainers see themselves as direct providers and few have as yet begun to embrace a broader view of training which looks critically at issues of planning and resource allocation. Many of the issues relating to HIV and AIDS that come up in local authorities do not always need a direct training course for staff. Much of the emphasis in HIV/AIDS training is on individual responses to the epidemic. It is rarely developmental, in the sense that it aims to measure and evaluate the individual's contribution to service and organisational goals.

Many authorities have embarked on wholesale programmes of staff training, and thousands of people are being trained or have been trained without detailed attention to their training needs or those of the organisation. Much training has been preceded by inadequate discussions with management, scant analysis of participants' work situations, and little attention to participants' learning needs and the learning process itself. Few attempts have been made to measure the outcomes of training – and few changes are made to courses in the light of what has been learned. Many HIV/AIDS training programmes are highly expensive exercises that cost authorities and government far more than the nominal cost of the trainers and the venue. It is worth noting though that some of these problems arise from a funding system in which there is pressure to spend the grants given, and in which grants are awarded on an annual rather than a longer-term basis. In this context, training can be an easy way out for a lethargic organisation.

Ideally, the evaluation of training programmes and responses should be located within its organisational setting.

Towards better practice

In order to progress, it is necessary to go back to basics. This involves identifying the difference between what people should know and do and what they actually do know and do. It also involves distinguishing more clearly macro considerations to do with the nature of the organisation and group behaviour change from micro concerns to do with individual training needs. By so doing, training responses can be better set against organisation values. Useful questions to ask here include:

- what is it that a particular department is trying to do in relation to HIV and AIDS?
- What does that same department want from its staff?
- Where are the staff now and where should they be in the future?
- How is this gap to be filled and monitored?

Some trainers also need to change the way they see what they do. Rarely do they see themselves as service providers. If they have a clearly articulated view, this is most usually in terms of their loyalty to individual participants or the course group. This primary contract leads inevitably to insufficient attention being paid to how the learning is being utilised and applied. It can also provide a kind of 'rationale' for trainers' lack of communication with managers. Thus the communication of findings from the evaluation carried out at the end of a workshop can be seen as an issue of 'confidentiality'. Course particants, too, may receive little feedback on their performance and there is the danger that they will initially overestimate the learning that has taken place. Yet training's true clients are, strictly speaking, not course participants but the organisation, its management and its clients.

HIV/AIDS training is not a unitary phenomenon with an agreed pattern and content. Service providers need training relating to their specific service areas; managers should be receiving training around the issues relating to their role as managers; and senior managers need training around the human resource management and personnel aspects of their work. Each group needs a different focus, and each a different course or form of training. If local authority trainers do not respond in this way they will not be allowing for the complexities associated with different needs. In order to move to this kind of situation, trainers will need to be trained themselves. They will have to grasp concepts that may at present be alien to them – predictors of future value, current performance indicators, realisable potential, ultimate value and cost-effectiveness measures. They will have to come to see themselves as 'trainers' first and foremost, not HIV/AIDS specialists.

Because existing approaches to evaluation rely so heavily on satisfaction criteria, HIV/AIDS trainers find it hard to respond to a researcher or an organisation's questions once they are posed. If this method of evaluation has to be used in the future then some attempt must be made to remove or minimise the subjective element by quantifying the information obtained. For example, descriptions could be assigned values and computed into overall scores applied across categories. In this way it could be possible to assign an overall learning score to each event. However, there are difficulties with this approach, especially when outcomes are evaluated by proxy or on the basis simply of what participants say. Ways need to be found of evaluating the effects of training on practice and evaluating how well skills, knowledge or understanding are retained. Throughout the research carried out in preparing *HIV Infection and AIDS: A Training Handbook for Local Authorities*, only one example of an attempt to assess the learning that had taken place on a course was found, and the trainers there indicated they were so shocked by what they found out that they decided not to follow the matter up!

Evaluation and assessment, however, can only be as effective as the organisation's capacity to use the data obtained. This is related both to the kind of information provided by the trainers and by the organisation's capacity to respond positively to what is found out. Current changes in local government are raising the profile of monitoring and evaluation in relation to services and the way in which they are provided. In the light of these new priorities, it is undeniably foolish for any organisation embarking on a major staff training exercise not to evaluate its effectiveness, and to do this trainers need to look wider than the event itself.

What is needed?

This final section will identify some of the things that are most needed if HIV/AIDS trainers in local authorities are to be able to respond positively to the challenges that face them. First, there is a need for a training programme for trainers or advisers. This should aim to help them decide what to evaluate and how to do it. As part of this training, participants should be encouraged to consider a broader role for themselves than that of teacher or instructor. Training is also needed in planning and in identifying monitoring and evaluation strategies that are predictive, rather than just descriptive. Trainers need guidance in identifying what is to be reviewed and how and when this is to take place. They also need help in identifying what to do with the information they collect.

Second, training plans should aim to assess the total value of the training system in social, as well as financial and learning, terms. Data should be systematically collected and analysed to improve learning and performance, and in order to provide feedback on the training activities. Third, local authorities themselves need to make some visible commitment to monitoring and evaluation. If they do this, HIV/AIDS trainers and advisers may be more encouraged to involve themselves in evaluation activities, with consequent spin-off for financial and budgetary control. As part of that commitment, local authorities should recognise, too, that effective evaluation takes time, energy and money. Once people realise that if evaluation does not take place then the costs will also be high, attitudes about evaluation can be changed. All training assumes transfer, and without evaluation and assessment there is no way to know if transfer has taken place.

There is, however, an inherent difficulty in evaluating training, in that the immediate results are often not easily demonstrable. The form of any review must address this issue. Effectiveness and value need to be understood in specific and demonstrable terms as well as in human resource terms. In order to do this it will be necessary to identify a number of predictors of the value of training activities. One way of doing this might be as shown in Figure 9:

*Figure 9 **Assessing the value of training activities***

1 **Current performance**	=		skills + knowledge + motivation (These can be assessed by systems of appraisal.)
2 **Potential**	= 1 +		capacity to be developed to improve performance, or enhance specialisation, or be prepared for new work etc.
3 **What is realisable**	= 2 +	+	opportunity for training support of management for transferring the learning into the workplace
4 **Value of the training** = 3 − 1			(This is the difference beween what is realisable and what the organisation and individual started with. It can be measured either in £s or in service terms to the organisation.)

Models also need to be developed to enable organisations and trainers to measure performance and attitudes in relation to the training objectives. The basis for one such model is shown in Figure 10.

*Figure 10 **Attitudes, performance and training objectives***

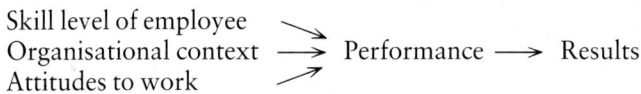

Skill level of employee
Organisational context ⟶ Performance ⟶ Results
Attitudes to work

Key attitudinal dimensions here could be self-attitude to the task, attitudes to others and attitudes to the organisation.

Decisions also need to be made as to whether outputs or outcomes are to be measured. Outputs could include having a training course itself and the number of trained persons that result from the course. Different kinds of outcomes that might be measured include individual outcomes, consequent outcomes and organisational outcomes. Additionally, it may be valuable to carry out a broad training audit involving detailed examination of every stage and aspect of the training process to see whether its design, implementation and evaluation have been adequately analysed at each stage.

Then there are issues of methodology to decide on in order to measure training gaps. Part of the problem here is that new research techniques may need to be developed, or existing ones modified, in order to assess training needs and identify training shortfalls. The scope of evaluation needs first to be determined. Planning and consultation are crucial if evaluation is to be a productive activity.

The major constraint stems from the fact that HIV/AIDS trainers do not yet have as much access as they need to mainstream training literature. As a result, they have largely avoided the challenge of developing a methodology and language for training analysis and evaluation. In the coming years, they cannot continue to take the need for training or the result of training as self-evident – this defensiveness may be understandable but it is shortsighted. Above all, it is essential that evaluation is not imposed by the organisation and management on their terms rather than those collectively agreed to by all sides. Intsead, everyone needs to be reminded of the benefits of evaluation and take on the challenge in an innovative and comprehensive way.

References

Clark, W. (1989) *HIV Infection and AIDS: A Training Handbook for Local Authorities.* London, Health Education Authority.

Jackson, T. (1988) Evaluation, Parts 1, 2, and 3. *Training and Development.* April, May, June.

CHAPTER SEVEN

Evaluating a Needle Exchange Scheme for Injecting Drug Users in Central London: Defining Success

Graham Hart

The primary function of needle and syringe exchange schemes for injecting drug users is to prevent the further spread of HIV infection. The major question facing those who would evaluate the efficacy of such schemes is, do they work? That is, are clients of needle exchange able to avoid HIV infection as a result of their appropriate use of the scheme? The final outcome measure appears deceptively straightforward – no new infections in the client population during the term of provision of the service. The most obvious and immediate means of ascertaining this is to use an HIV-antibody test on all, or at least a representative sample, of clients, repeatedly over time. In addition, in order to determine accurately the efficacy of the scheme, it would be necessary also to test a representative sample of non-attenders during the same period. If the rate of infection in this control group was greater than in the client population then a causal link between attendance at the scheme and its protective effect in relation to HIV infection could be demonstrated, or at least posited. Such a model of clinical epidemiological investigation is not always possible to practice, however, for reasons which will become clear when a real evaluation of a needle exchange scheme in central London is described here.

In this chapter, one HIV-related service for drug users will be described, and an account given of the methods used to monitor and evaluate this service. An attempt will also be made to look critically at the approach taken, and suggestions made as to ways in which future research could build upon experience gained so far, particularly in the use of complimentary methods.

The context

In September 1987, the Middlesex Hospital opened its needle exchange scheme at 16A Cleveland Street, London W1, formerly the hospital's

Department of Surgical Appliances. A needle and syringe exchange scheme had been offered previously in the Accident and Emergency (A & E) Department of University College Hospital (UCH), but with the provision of financial support from the Department of Health it had been possible to dedicate premises to an experimental service. Staffed in the first instance by two drug and health education workers, Cleveland Street soon proved popular with users in central London, partly because of its location close to the major drug dealing subculture in the Charing Cross Road/Soho area, and partly because of the positive attitudes of its staff to clients.

In agreeing to provide 'pump priming' funding the Department of Health stipulated that the scheme be incorporated in a national evaluation of the effectiveness of needle exchange initiatives. This was agreed, and Cleveland Street became one of the exchanges to be monitored by Stimson and his team of researchers (the Monitoring Research Group) at Goldsmiths' College, University of London (see Stimson *et al*, 1988). This involved the professionals working in the agencies specified completing 'intake sheets' on each client, recording basic demographic data and drug histories, and more detailed interviews with clients willing to participate approximately one month and three to four months after first attendance. These were conducted variously by agency and research staff.

Involvement in this research occurred as a result of previous work with drug users at the Drug Dependency Unit in the same district, Bloomsbury Health Authority. In a study of clients of this service it had been found that the major reason given by drug users for the sharing of needles and syringes was unavailability of injecting equipment at the time of use, and therefore the necessity for use of another drug user's 'works' (Hart, Sonnex, Petherick *et al*, 1989). Interest developed in the possibility of increasing the availability of sterile needles and syringes to injecting drug users in the district, and of measuring the effectivenes of such an intervention. An initial request was therefore made for Department of Health funding of a dedicated needle exchange scheme. This led to the setting up of 'The Exchange'.

Wishing to continue an involvement in this area of enquiry, but not wishing to duplicate the research efforts of the Monitoring Research Group (MRG) at Goldsmiths' College, an application was made to the AIDS Education and Research Trust (AVERT) to fund a two-year project to generate data which could be used by the MRG, but which would also complement its work and add to the literature in the area. Issues of particular interest included the last occasion of sharing needles and syringes, and the use of other drug, medical and social services locally. However, the major addition to the research protocol was the use of a salivary antibody test for HIV which, it was hoped, would provide some indication of the extent to which attendance at

The Exchange had some protective effect for clients in avoiding HIV infection during the period of their use of the scheme. The results of this study will be described presently, but first a more detailed account will be given of the purpose of this monitoring and the particular techniques used.

The research agenda

To claim that the ideal form of research on the efficacy of needle exchange in preventing HIV infection would involve the use of HIV-antibody tests, over time, on the client population and a 'control' group of demographically and behaviourally comparable injecting drug users is to simplify the many research questions that the provision of such a service raises. To reduce these to one single issue is to do a gross injustice to the providers of such a service and to its clients. Apart from questions of behavioural change, one would also wish to collect attitudinal data in relation to the service offered, to HIV and to AIDS, as well as information – from clients, service providers and other local drug professionals – on the place of needle exchange in the broader context of statutory and non-statutory drugs services in the district. Research methods would include the collection of qualitative as well as survey-based quantitative data, and the aim would be fully to elucidate the contribution of needle and syringe exchange to the improved health and social welfare of clients.

Exigencies of research funding, however, and in particular the limits on resources, time and personnel, mean that research questions often have to be restricted to what is most immediately achievable. Apart from limited research findings which posited an association between the provision of needle and syringe exchange in Amsterdam (van den Hoek *et al*, 1989) and in Sydney (Wolk *et al*, 1988) with reduced incidence of HIV-antibody infection in the communities served, at the time that the research described here began, no firm data on the changes in the HIV-antibody status of attenders at such schemes were available. It was therefore felt that the most pressing question in 1987/8 related to the public health function of the schemes in preventing new infections. Although this was a self-imposed research agenda, national and international interest in needle exchange is primarily centred on this issue, and it was felt appropriate to report on data from this aspect of the work as soon as possible (Hart, Carvell, Woodward *et al*, 1989).

It was subsequently possible to address some of the other questions that the provision of this service raises, most notably its contribution to improved general health in clients, the integration of the service with others directed towards drug users locally, and the overall operating philosophy of the staff in terms of the broader function of needle

interview is available. People who were approached and repeatedly refused to participate were not counted; this is unfortunate, as this statistic would have provided a better sense of the acceptability of the research to the target population. On the basis of data available, in terms of sex, age, age at first daily injection, recent frequency of injecting and sharing behaviour, there were no significant differences between all attenders and the sample who were interviewed, so there can be confidence that the study group is representative of attenders generally. Nevertheless, response rate is important and should be recorded.

The findings

This section will offer a brief résumé of the study's major findings. Essentially, the scheme proved popular with clients, with an average of 257 injecting drug users attending The Exchange every month of the year of study. Moreover, compliance, in terms of returning used syringes, has been high (see above) and there was no increase in injecting during the study, thus refuting the claim that drug use among attenders would increase. Comparing the year prior to their entry to the scheme to recent sharing behaviour, a reduction in the levels of lending and borrowing injecting equipment among clients was found, and a further reduction in sharing was demonstrated in those who were re-interviewed three to four months after first joining the scheme. Clients' sexual behaviour did not change substantially, but there was a high prevalence of condom use compared to other mainly heterosexual populations, and very frequent condom use among those with multiple sexual partners. During the year of study, we found that 7 of 121 at first test were HIV-antibody positive (6%); a further two clients became HIV-antibody positive on the second test, giving a prevalence for the year of 9 of 121 (7%). It was not possible to determine whether the two clients whose HIV-antibody status changed had been at risk prior to or after their entry to the scheme. These data are fully reported in Hart, Carvell, Woodward et al (1989).

We also found that The Exchange functioned as a referral agency, putting clients into contact with other drug, health and social services locally. During the first 18 months of the scheme's life, 277 individuals received and took up 510 referrals to other services, demonstrating that The Exchange, as a low threshold access service, was well linked to a network of caring agencies in the statutory and non-statutory sectors. Further information on this aspect of the study can be found in Carvell and Hart (1990).

Details of the development of drug and other HIV-related services in Bloomsbury Health District, including needle exchange, can be found in George and Hart (in Pye et al, 1989), and the place of needle exchange in the British historical response to drug use is explored in Chapter 11 of Aggleton *et al* (1990). The operating philosophy of the scheme's staff and the communication strategies employed with clients are described in Hart, Woodward and Carvell *et al* (1989).

Building upon experience: lessons learned

It has been stressed that this study had limited aims and, for the most part, these have been fulfilled. The major problem with undertaking research into a new service such a needle exchange, however, lies in defining the meaning of success. For example, although it was hoped to focus on behavioural change and incidence of HIV infection, for the workers in the agency many more issues were significant to them. Was the service doing as much as it could, and being delivered appropriately? Were messages regarding harm minimisation (a cornerstone of needle exchange philosophy) getting across to clients, and being put into practice? For others, however, the major questions to ask of needle exchange have yet to be answered, and its success is far from demonstrated. As we undertook no interviews with, or saliva testing of, a comparable group of non-attenders we cannot say finally that it is the needle exchange programme which is helping to keep the level of HIV infection in London relatively low. This might have occurred as a result of health education to drug users, or simply because of changes in the subculture of injectors which would have occurred regardless of the presence of needle exchange schemes.

Certain lessons regarding monitoring and evaluating this needle exchange programme have been learned as a result of undertaking this study, and these are worth discussing briefly. As the service was new, and the staff uncertain as to the continuing appeal of The Exchange, the workers were concerned that monitoring and evaluation should inconvenience the clients as little as possible. This meant that the ideal method of measuring HIV-antibody prevalence – testing as many clients as possible during a short period of time, and repeating this at a later date to measure any change – was not considered possible. In fact this was subsequently done in January 1990, but at a time when the scheme was firmly established and the workers had fewer worries about the acceptability of such an intervention. It is debatable, and finally indeterminable, whether in fact such a design would not always have been acceptable to clients, and whether the natural concerns of the drug workers properly to establish the service prior to any major research intervention reflected their own fears and anxieties rather than those of clients about the service. Maintaining the goodwill and support of the professionals working in the agency, however, is as important to good research outcomes as not offending clients, and it was preferable to accede to the views of the staff on this issue rather than threaten the whole monitoring and evaluation exercise.

The research assistant working on the study spent the majority of her time in The Exchange recruiting clients to the study, interviewing and undertaking routine administration as part of the monitoring of the service. This more than filled her working day, but there were also opportunities here to undertake some qualitative work with the client group. For example, aspects of the subculture of central London users and their interactions with the police, statutory agency workers and, of course, other drug users and dealers would have been worth recording and describing. This would not have compromised other aspects of the study, although it is recognised that further resources would have been required if every aspect of the study were to be fully analysed and written up. Such enquiry would not merely have been of academic interest, since information of this kind could prove invaluable in understanding the social pressures towards certain types of risk behaviour for HIV infection, and in monitoring the role of peer groups and others in changes in the drug-using community.

One potential criticism mentioned earlier concerned the effect of the provision of needle exchange on all drug users in the area served, and the need to interview and test a comparable sample of non-attenders. That there are many problems associated with such work – particularly collecting blood or saliva samples for laboratory testing in the street or cafés, and keeping these safe and under conditions which are not detrimental to the researcher or the sample – is no valid reason for not attempting such an exercise. Interviews have certainly been conducted under such circumstances, and participant observation is a recognised and accepted method of recording data (Power, 1989). Again, however, there are resource and staffing implications here, and research funding bodies must be persuaded of the value of such an exercise. Unlike agency-based work, where the researcher's presence can become accepted and expected, street-based work is far less comfortable. It can also be dangerous, particularly when it involves the study of illicit activity. It is also less predictable in terms of the amount of data it will generate.

Research does not take place in a vacuum, and researchers must take note of and learn from others working in the same or similar fields. Many of the strategies described above have been used in other cities and countries and have proved their worth (see Hart, 1989). However, at the time this study was designed and funded, more limited goals were pursued and, we hope, achieved. Research in The Exchange, and other needle exchange schemes, continues and we intend to learn from, and build upon, the experience gained so far.

Implications for policy and practice

The research undertaken at The Exchange has been useful, at local, national and, to a certain extent, international levels. Locally, findings regarding the risk behaviours of attenders at the scheme have been noted and acted upon by the agency's workers. For example, those who have found it impossible under certain circumstances to avoid sharing needles and syringes have now been provided with specially designed bleach bottles and information on how to clean needles and syringes to a standard that would substantially reduce the risk of contracting or transmitting HIV were the virus present and 'works' shared. Local workers are also aware of findings regarding safer sexual behaviour, and the need to continue to encourage and facilitate this in clients at risk through sexual contact. This is a fast-moving field, however, and new initiatives introduced by agency workers invariably run ahead of research findings; nevertheless, the research findings have contributed to further development in the agency.

Also at the local level, but outside the immediate confines of The Exchange, the research has a contribution to make in relation to the continued funding of the agency. Initial funding for the scheme from the Department of Health was short-lived, and it was expected that in due course the district health authority would take over the costs of staff and equipment. The district did do this, using money from its HIV/AIDS budget, and did so prior to the appearance of any firm findings from the research. However, with tight budgets generally for all health services, and particularly preventive and community-based projects, it cannot be assumed that this level of funding will continue indefinitely. The findings of the study will contribute substantially to medical audit, and may play a role in encouraging managers to continue supporting the scheme.

At a national level, and at the time the study was undertaken, there were few studies of anti-HIV prevalence in drug-using populations; data have therefore proved useful in the monitoring of the development of the HIV epidemic in the country. The methodology employed has also been recognised as a valuable means of collecting data on a population not easily studied, and in particular the acceptability to injecting drug users of the non-invasive technique of saliva sampling has meant that studies are now planned or under way which will extend our understanding of the epidemiology of HIV in Britain. At a service level, our reports on the organisation and functioning of the scheme may prove useful to those planning similar services in other health districts, although we would not wish to be prescriptive about a model of health care which, though appropriate for this particular client group, may not suit injecting drug users in other parts of the country.

Finally, at an international level, research reports have been published in internationally respected and recognised journals, and papers given at national and international conferences. Requests for reprints of publications have come from countries with few or no needle exchange schemes but with drug problems, and, when the findings have been presented, substantial interest has been expressed by people who wish to prevent further HIV infection in their drug-using population. This is, however, just one study among many that have taken or are taking place, and it would be wrong to suggest that it alone has influenced attitudes to the provision of such a service. However, as part of a growing literature in the area, it has contributed to the debates about the efficacy of needle exchange, and in particular has provided firm evidence that this can be a safe public health intervention.

In this chapter, one approach to the study of needle exchange has been described, in one district and serving a particular client population of long-term, older and predominantly male injecting drug users. While this methodology has proved useful in central London, in other districts with different populations and problems it may not be suitable. It is not possible easily to export this model to other areas without first understanding the type and extent of drug use in each area. Local circumstances demand local responses, both at the level of service provision and in the approaches taken in measuring the efficacy of new interventions. Were the evaluation and monitoring of the service to begin again – in the light of hindsight and with experience of similar studies – changes would be made in its design and execution. Nevertheless, in offering this as one way of researching a needle exchange, and in discussing some alternative or complementary approaches, the hope is that those considering setting up and evaluating needle exchange may benefit from experience gained so far.

References

Aggleton, P.J., Davies, P. and Hart, G.J. (Eds.) (1990) *AIDS: Individual, Cultural and Policy Dimensions.* Basingstoke, Falmer Press.

Carvell, A.L.M. and Hart, G.J. (1990) Help-seeking and referrals in a needle exchange: a comprehensive service to injecting drug users. *British Journal of Addiction*, 85, 235–40.

Hart, G.J. (1989) Editorial: Injecting drug use, HIV and AIDS. *AIDS Care*, 1, 237–45.

Hart, G.J., Carvell, A.L.M., Woodward, N., *et al* (1989) Evaluation of needle exchange in central London: behaviour change and anti-HIV status over one year. *AIDS*, 3, 261–5.

Hart, G.J., Sonnex, C., Petherick, A., *et al* (1989) Risk behaviours for HIV infection among injecting drug users attending a drug dependency clinic. *British Medical Journal*, **298**, 1081–3.

Hart, G.J., Woodward N. and Carvell, A. (1989) Needle exchange in central London: operating philosophy and communication strategies. *AIDS Care*, **2**, 125–34.

Johnson, A.M., Parry, J.V., Best, S.J., *et al* (1988) HIV surveillance by testing saliva. *AIDS*, **2**, 369–71.

Parry, J.V., Perry, K.R. and Mortimer, P.P. (1987) Sensitive assays for viral antibody in saliva: an alternative to tests on serum. *Lancet*, **ii**, 72–5.

Power, R. (1989) Participant observation and its place in the study of drug abuse. *British Journal of Addiction*, **84**, 43–52.

Pye, M., Kapila, M., Buckley, G. and Cunningham, D. (Eds.) (1989) *Responding to the AIDS Challenge*. London, Health Education Authority/Longman.

Stimson, G.V., Alldritt, L.J., Dolan, K.A., Donoghoe, M.C. and Lart, R.A. (1988) *Injecting Equiment Exchange Schemes: Final Report*. London, Goldsmiths' College.

van den Hoek, J.A.R., van Haastrecht, H.J.A. and Coutinho, R.A. (1989) Risk reduction among intravenous drug users in Amsterdam under the influence of AIDS. *American Journal of Public Health*, **79**, 1355–7.

Wolk, J.J., Wodak, A., Morlet, A. *et al* (1988) Syringe HIV seroprevalence and behavioural and demographic characteristics of intravenous drug users in Sydney, Australia, 1987. *AIDS*, **2**, 247–54.

CHAPTER EIGHT

An Economic Approach to the Evaluation of HIV/AIDS Health Education Programmes

Christine Godfrey and Keith Tolley

One of the initial responses to the threat of HIV/AIDS was to devote considerable resources to mass media health education programmes. Between March 1986 and November 1987 a total of £22.5m was provided by the Department of Health for newspaper, television and leaflet campaigns. Education and other prevention measures were seen as the only method of curtailing the spread of HIV. Local initiatives were encouraged through the use of earmarked funds from 1988/9 to each Regional Health Authority in England and to Health Boards in Scotland. It has, however, proved difficult to ensure that a substantial proportion of the earmarked funding goes to prevention rather than treatment. The difficulty of demonstrating the effectiveness of education and other prevention programmes, in this as in other areas related to health behaviour, is one of the factors which may influence the allocation of funds. The pressure to demonstrate effectivenes is likely to grow in the immediate future, not least because recent estimates of the incidence of the HIV infection have been lower than earlier predictions (PHLS, 1990).

Economists have long advocated a number of techniques to assess the costs and benefits of different health programmes, although many activities of the health service remain poorly evaluated from an economic point of view. In this chapter, some of the issues that may arise in applying these techniques to the evaluation of programmes of HIV/AIDS education are examined. In the first section, the types of questions that may be addressed by economic evaluations are discussed and the general principles of such studies are outlined. Some of the different costs and benefits which could be included in the evaluation of HIV/AIDS health promotion/disease prevention programmes are considered in the second section. Because a number of economists have outlined the problems that can occur with inadequate evaluation, in the third section a checklist of questions which may help guide practical evaluations is considered. Finally, some concluding remarks are made on the advantages and disadvantages of an economic approach to the evaluation of HIV/AIDS health education programmes.

Issues in economic evaluation

There are a number of different types of economic evaluation. The choice of technique to evaluate a particular prevention activity depends on the policy questions which those proposing the evaluation seek to address. In some cases a very wide perspective may be taken and the worth of undertaking an HIV/AIDS programme compared to a completely different activity, for example building a road, may be sought. More often, particularly in the light of recent health service and local government reforms, the question of the value for money devoted to HIV/AIDS compared to other health or social care is being raised. To some extent the government, by earmarking funds, has sheltered existing programmes from wider evaluations of this kind, although these earmarked funds were only intended to be part of the total funds devoted to the prevention and treatment of this disease. Another type of policy question involves the appropriate distribution of funds within the HIV/AIDS budget, and in particular the balance between prevention, treatment and research. Finally, there are questions of priorities within the prevention budget which will include choices of approach, e.g. mass media or local campaigns, the issue of targeting, and the efficiency of particular campaigns and the agencies involved in the programme. Frequently a number of agencies have been jointly involved in local HIV/AIDS initiatives. For example, in Lothian the planning and providing of a safer-sex roadshow involved the health board, the local authority and the voluntary sector. There are particular problems in evaluating the myriad schemes that may originate in, or may be located within, the voluntary sector.

Cost-benefit analyses

The purpose of economic evaluations of alternative policies is to identify which options give the best value for the resources expended. The scope of the alternative policies under consideration gives a guide to the range of both costs and benefits that need to be evaluated, and hence the type of economic evaluation to be undertaken. The most general questions require a whole range of costs and benefits to be measured in some common unit, usually money, to allow comparisons to be made. Hence *cost-benefit* analyses are used to compare, say, a health promotion scheme to a road building scheme, where the aim would be to determine which scheme gives the greatest net benefit. There are, however, difficulties in putting money values on some intangible benefits and in particular putting a monetary value on life itself.

Cost-effectiveness studies

For more limited questions, and where the output from the competing programmes being considered are similar, *cost-effectiveness* studies may be undertaken. In health evaluations this technique has been used to examine the costs and benefits of different medical interventions on the basis of the cost per life year saved/gained from treatment. Clearly more specific measures could be used if other outcomes between the programmes are the same. Targets for different needle exchange schemes may be evaluated in this framework having, for example, as the effectiveness measure, the number of injecting drug users using the scheme or the numbers of needles exchanged. The disadvantage of such cost-effectiveness studies (and the limited and specific measurement of programme outcomes) is that comparisons with the use of resources in other activities cannot be drawn from the results of such evaluations. For example, it would clearly not be possible to compare the results of the evaluation of two needle exchange schemes with those of other types of prevention or education programmes aimed at injecting drug users if a specific effectiveness measure such as the number of needles exchanged had been used.

Cost-utility analyses

Both cost-effectiveness and cost-benefit analyses have disadvantages for health evaluations. In particular there have been problems in devising adequate measures of health care outcomes which reflect both the quantity of life (often the only factor considered in a cost-effectiveness analysis) and the quality of life. Putting monetary values on life, which could in theory encompass both quantity and quality, has always been considered problematic, and many of the ways in which such values have been obtained have been criticised (Drummond, 1980). Hence health economists carrying out *cost-utility analyses* have attempted to devise measures such as QALYs or Well-Years which reflect the utility or satisfaction gained from changes in health states (Drummond *et al*, 1987). These measures are still being developed and evaluated and there is much debate about their use in the evaluation of health education programmes (Cribb and Haycox, 1989).

Whatever the technique chosen, economic evaluations have a number of features in common, and undertaking such a study involves considering the inputs, process and outcomes of the competing policies (Figure 11). This involves identifying, measuring and valuing the resources consumed in health promotion and the health promotion activity itself, plus those of the competing, alternative policies. There will always be some policy alternative, even if this involves doing nothing.

Figure 11 *The nature of economic evaluation*

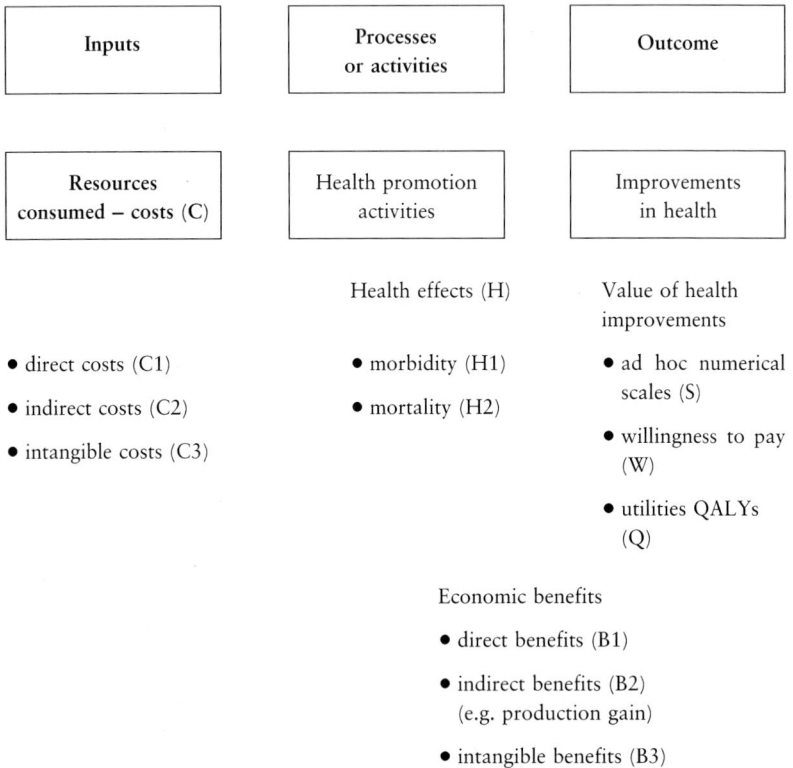

Inputs	Processes or activities	Outcome
Resources consumed – costs (C)	Health promotion activities	Improvements in health

	Health effects (H)	Value of health improvements
• direct costs (C1)	• morbidity (H1)	• ad hoc numerical scales (S)
• indirect costs (C2)	• mortality (H2)	
• intangible costs (C3)		• willingness to pay (W)
		• utilities QALYs (Q)

Economic benefits

• direct benefits (B1)

• indirect benefits (B2)
  (e.g. production gain)

• intangible benefits (B3)

Adapted from Torrance (1986)

Costs and benefits in HIV/AIDS education programmes

Inputs and costs

Whatever the type of economic evaluation being undertaken, the inputs and costs of the programme need to be considered. Valuing and measuring the direct inputs to a programme may be considered the simplest part of the evaluation, especially as many HIV/AIDS prevention/education initiatives have used specific new earmarked funds. However, there may be hidden costs, such as the use of existing staff, or overvalued resources, such as an unused office which had no or little alternative use. Values used in economic costings refer to the best alternative use of resources or their *opportunity cost*. Hence, even if staff involved in a new programme were previously employed by the health service or local authority, so that there are no extra items of cost in financial terms on the balance sheet, the time of these staff could have been spent in some alternative way. The value of this alternative use of time should be considered in an economic evaluation. Problems can occur, however, in determining costs of programmes when resources, both capital and labour, are shared between a number of programmes. It may also be difficult to identify the opportunity costs of voluntary services or of initiatives to introduce health education topics more generally in the media, for example in current affairs programmes or in 'soap' story-lines.

Some costs may fall on agencies other than the one initiating the programme. This may be by design, for example when joint initiatives are undertaken, or when a national or local campaign generates extra work for health and other professionals in giving advice and passing on campaign material. Economic evaluations are usually conducted from a society-wide perspective, and such costs would be included as part of the study, even though they might not fall on the pro-gramme budget. This clearly separates economic from financial appraisals. For policy-makers, however, there may be some requirement in presenting evaluations to outline where costs are borne as well as any total figure.

Costs may also fall on individuals participating in the health education programme. An examination of the tangible and intangible costs which may be incurred by individuals can provide insight into the different success rates of alternative schemes. In particular, it may highlight problems of access, perhaps in terms of distance travelled or inappropriate opening hours of those initiatives which require some participation (for example a needle exchange scheme) or the inaccessibility of language for health education material. Other costs falling on individuals could include factors such as the anxiety involved in undertaking a blood test. There are clear difficulties in measuring intangible items such as these, and they have been ignored in many evaluations. While precise measurement may be difficult, it may, however, be possible to give some idea of how such costs vary between the alternative policies under consideration.

Health education programmes may also generate a number of indirect costs. These include demands for screening tests and counselling which may follow an educational campaign. If these costs are underestimated, or follow-up inquiries cannot be dealt with because of inadequate resources, then the impact of a particular campaign may be severely curtailed. It should be noted that there are a number of costs and benefits associated with HIV-antibody testing. These include the costs to the individuals of being identified as being HIV-positive in terms of difficulties in obtaining insurance and employment as well as the possible wider social benefits from changes in behaviour which may limit the spread of the virus (Rovira, 1990a). The balance of costs and benefits to the individual of testing may change given that there is some evidence of the efficacy of Zidovudine in cases of asymptomatic HIV infection.

Health promotion activities and processes

Much of the information which is routinely available within health and local services relates to process, rather than outcome, measures. It is important in evaluations to consider the process of the education/ prevention programme as separate from the outcomes. Insights into the efficiency of the process may be gained from such studies, even though the most efficient process could not be deemed worthwhile if outcomes were unchanged or small in relation to costs. Lessons can be learned from retrospective evaluations, other HIV/AIDS campaigns or other areas of health education. If, however, these programmes have not been fully evaluated, or the evaluations are not readily available, many resources could be wasted. Policy responses to HIV/AIDS have been varied and early schemes have many elements of experimentation. Clearly such 'new' schemes have an element of cost due to their innovatory character. By studying the process of the activity it should be possible to separate out the costs of the experimental element.

Objectives and outcomes

In Figure 11 the benefits of health educational programmes are seen in terms of health. The nature of HIV/AIDS suggests that the largest benefit of a prevention programme is the potential saving of life. Others have argued, however, that having information is of value in itself, whether or not it is used to change behaviour, because informed choices can be made (Cohen and Henderson, 1988). Another view concerning the importance of health education programmes suggests that they can play a more complex role in the policy-making process (Harrison and Tether, 1990). Campaigns about the serious public health implications of HIV/AIDS may be thought necessary to generate support for the transfer of resources from other activities. Alternatively, a health education campaign may be viewed by governments and administrators a being a 'visible response' to a difficult social problem, and, therefore, a source of political, rather than health, benefits. This is an area of debate, but the issue may be determined by the objectives of the policy-maker and the type of programme being evaluated. For example, if a policy-maker was primarily concerned with increasing knowledge, then alternative programmes could be evaluated to find the most cost-effective means of achieving this objective. Within such evaluations, economists may suggest there could be additional benefits (such as prolonging life) which vary between programmes. This source of information could be used in the decision-making process, but it is ultimately the policy-maker who decides the objectives of policy and the weights given to different outcomes.

A recent survey of local statutory sector HIV/AIDS programmes indicates that a wide variety of programmes has been initiated by health and local authorities but few authorities have been explicit about the objectives (Beardshaw et al, 1990). The Oxford Regional Health Authority's draft policy would seem to be the exception in suggesting that the aim is to change behaviour and not just to educate or inform. Six specific target areas were set out in this draft policy. These targets may be considered intermediate objectives, the primary outcome being a reduction in new cases of HIV infection. They do, however, provide a set of indicators that could theoretically be measured. The areas identified were:

- a reduction of sexual partners
- the adoption of safer sex practices
- condom use for penetrative sex
- the avoidance of drug injection
- the use of clean equipment where drug injection is practised
- developing understanding, compassion and tolerance towards people with HIV/AIDS.

Objectives of many other programmes were far more general, being concerned with raising awareness about AIDS and HIV, either in the whole population or in certain subgroups. It is also clear that most authorities devoted a large part of their resources for HIV/AIDS education to staff training. This training had a wider purpose than changing risky personal behaviour of staff, although the health service and local authorities are large employers and workplace schemes are one means of reaching a sizeable proportion of the population. For those who are most likely to come into contact with people with HIV there was a need to institute measures to stop the spread of the disease, allay unnecessary anxiety about how the virus is transmitted and educate those from whom the general population are likely to seek information. It is important to recognise that staff training schemes have different objectives from a programme to educate the general population, and this needs to be reflected in the measurement of the expected outcomes.

Identifying and measuring outcomes

By setting out the objectives of different policies, and by identifying the different types of costs and benefits associated with each, an economic approach to evaluation can be employed. As with costs, it is usual to adopt a society-wide perspective when identifying and measuring outcomes. HIV/AIDS has a wide range of effects for individuals, be they infected or not, as well as for non-health agencies and the economy. Not all campaigns will be designed to affect all possible outcomes, and it is important to identify which outcomes each campaign seeks to influence.

From a health perspective, one of the major benefits that may be expected of prevention/education programmes is the saving of lives. Currently, the number of people who have died as a result of AIDS is still small relative to other causes. The cumulative number of deaths is now forecast to be in the region of 6380 by 1993 (PHLS, 1990). This forecast, which is rather lower than that made two or three years ago, in part reflects changing behaviour, particularly among gay men. From an economic perspective, quantity of life is also important, and here it is important to recognise that there are differences in the ranking of potential benefits from changing disease patterns if an indicator of life years lost is used, rather than the numbers of deaths (Godfrey et al, 1989). AIDS is associated with the deaths of predominantly young people, and calculations for France show the large demographic impact the disease can have. It is calculated that in 1989 the loss of life years from AIDS was similar to that associated with infectious disease or alcohol psychosis, and by 1991 will be associated with 8.9 per cent of the total life years lost of those dying before the age of 65, an amount similar to the calculations for suicide and motor vehicle accidents (Guiguet and Valleron, 1990). While the UK has lower reported rates of HIV/AIDS than France, the impact of the disease is likely to increase dramatically in the next few years.

Improving the quality of life of those diagnosed with HIV is another important potential outcome, especially if some comparisons are to be made to non-HIV/AIDS-related prevention or treatment. HIV/AIDS involves pain and distress for those affected as well as for relatives and friends, although positive aspects of lifestyle, such as an improvement in diet and health maintenance, should not be discounted. Many of the costs which affect the quality of life of those who have HIV/AIDS are not, however, health-related and arise from discrimination in the labour or housing markets. These aspects would not necessarily be considered in a clinical evaluation, and Maynard (1990) suggests that a whole range of evaluations could be considered involving an examination of labour, housing and social care. Some health education programmes could be directed at reducing discrimination by changing society's attitudes to those who have HIV/AIDS, and their successful evaluation might involve measures of changes in the quality of life or the ability to function within the community without resorting to high cost hospital care.

Health education programmes may have a number of other outcomes with benefit (or costs) that should be evaluated. At the time of the first mass media campaign there was concern expressed about the 'worried well'. If scare campaigns have only a limited effect on behaviour, but succeed in worrying a large number of individuals at low risk of infection, then costs could outweigh benefits. However, there may also be general health and social benefits derived from education campaigns which correct misinformation, for example, on how the virus is transmitted. And if behaviour is changed, there may be additional health benefits from lower levels of sexually transmitted diseases in general, or injecting drug use. These are some of the potental indirect benefits of an educational programme.

Health costs

Treatments for HIV/AIDS are expensive, and a saving of health care costs can be seen as one of the benefits of HIV/AIDS health education. Individual estimates of the cost of treatment have varied, but unit costs per patient year in Oxfordshire have recently been estimated at between £14,000 and £17,000 (Rees, 1990). More generally, the Department of Health has announced earmarked funding for hospital and community services of £126m for 1990/1 in England and Wales (a 5 per cent increase on the amount received by each authority in the previous year). In addition there has been a substantial increase in the direct grant for social care funding, for which social service departments in England have to bid, to nearly £10m for the same year. These departments are expected to meet a minimum of 30 per cent of the expenditure on HIV/AIDS social care from their mainstream budgets (Tolley and Maynard, 1990). This earmarking of some funds makes it easier to determine the annual cost of medical care, social care and prevention for HIV/AIDS than for other diseases, but it should be noted that, when it comes to an economic evaluation of health education programmes, the relevant cost would be expected *savings* on health care expenditures. This calculation would require some anticipation of the future costs of treatment (which are uncertain) and the calculation of the change in the lifetime health and social care costs for individuals who die prematurely (Rovira, 1990a).

One of the indirect costs of illness considered in some studies is the level of production losses associated with sickness or premature deaths. Using the loss of labour as a resource as a sole valuation of loss of life has been criticised, and it is arguable whether such effects should be considered *in addition* to the valuation of the quality and quantity of life which would take place within a cost-utility study. However, further infections could have a number of effects on the economies of some countries because of demographic effects, strains on some services, and effects on activities such as tourism. The effect of HIV/AIDS on the social system as a whole is difficult to measure and is outside the scope of most economic evaluations.

Value judgements, affected by social attitudes, are involved in costing studies, and it is therefore especially important to state clearly what assumptions are being made and to test the sensitivity of results to changes in these assumptions. Social values may be particularly important when considering equity or distribution questions. O'Brien (1990) examines these equity issues in relation to targeting campaigns towards some groups such as injecting drug users.

Linking outcome measures with programmes

Several different outcomes of changing the pattern of the spread of the virus have been outlined. There remain, however, problems in attempting to link changes in any of these outcomes to specific health education programmes. A necessary step is to model the relationship between changes in behaviour and the incidence of HIV infection. In the past, this modelling has been difficult because of lack of knowledge about the disease and its transmission, and lack of information about risky behaviour. Epidemiological models of the process of transmission have since improved, although knowledge about risk behaviour is still sparse. Large-scale sexual behaviour studies in Britain have been constrained by a lack of government approval, and hence funding. Anonymous testing will be a valuable aid in charting the spread of the virus. Given the remaining uncertainties, scenario analyses could play a useful role in evaluation by providing a range of estimates linked to different assumptions (Rovira, 1990b).

Even if some attempts can be made to chart the relationship between changes in behaviour and the health outcomes, this does not solve the problem of attributing changes to particular educational programmes. Studies involving baseline surveys, control groups and adequate follow-ups are necessary for isolating effects of this kind. Even these types of evaluation, however, may fail to measure the cumulative effect of a series of educational campaigns and media attention. Engleman and Forbes (1984) in a review of the economic aspects of health education suggest that 'failure to identify programme effects using inappropriate methods of evaluation should not be misinterpreted as providing evidence of programme failure'. Moreover, single programmes cannot be expected to meet all goals or to produce immediate outcomes. Some types of education programmes may pose problems for evaluation and the pattern of both costs and benefits would be expected to vary between mass media campaigns and specific local initiatives. A willingness to evaluate may, however, increase the chances of funding for health educational programmes of all descriptions.

It should be noted that the considerable amount of research that is needed to provide reliable estimates of risk behaviour and to develop scenario analyses is outside the scope and resources of many locally based programmes. There are therefore some developments in the methodology of economic evaluation of HIV/AIDS programmes that need to be undertaken centrally, along with the task of collating and disseminating information from local evaluations themselves.

Evaluating the evaluations

Several problems can occur with inadequate economic evaluations and various checklists have been developed to evaluate existing economic studies (see, for example, Drummond *et al*, 1987). This is especially important when the results from evaluations from past programmes are being used to decide on future priorities. It is necessary, for example, to ask questions about the objectives of the appraisal. If a narrow focus has been taken, then the generality of the results for future planning may be restricted. Evaluations may also be limited if some possible alternative policies have not been considered. Specific steps in judging how health care costs and benefits have been identified, measured and valued have been outlined (Drummond *et al*, 1987). Other questions include issues of discounting, marginal analyses and the sensitivity of results to particular assumptions. Economic theory suggests that future costs and benefits are not valued as highly as those occurring in the present time period, and the issue of discounting benefits is particularly important for determining the results of the evaluation of health education programmes. Marginality involves examining questions about the additional cost of acquiring additional benefits. For example, bringing about change in the behaviour of some groups may be relatively expensive. Finally sensitivity analyses are particularly important because there is so much uncertainty about the range and size of different outcomes.

Conclusions

There is no single answer to the question of how an economic evaluation of a particular HIV/AIDS education programme should be carried out. There are several different costing techniques. The choice of method, and consequently the costs and benefits which need to be measured, will vary according to the nature of the evaluation exercise and the objectives of the programme being considered. Available evidence on the effectiveness of prevention or treatment programmes has not been considered in this chapter, and there are considerable gaps in our knowledge. These make it difficult to determine the appropriate level of resources that should be devoted to HIV/AIDS; to decide how resources should be divided between prevention, treatment or research; to make decisions about if, or how, programmes should be targeted; and to identify the best methods for delivering health education. Information from well-conducted evaluation studies will be required to fill these gaps and to develop answers to these questions.

In conclusion, it can be said that the general frameworks and checklists that economists have developed in other areas can be used to test the usefulness of existing studies in the field of HIV/AIDS education evaluation. A number of key issues, both practical and theoretical, remain to be resolved, however, and future work will need to address these with some urgency if economists and others are to play an effective role in evaluating HIV/AIDS education programmes.

Acknowledgements

The authors would like to thank the Economic and Social Research Council and the Department of Health for financial support and Mike Drummond and Ken Wright for helpful comments on an earlier version of the paper.

References

Beardshaw V., Hunter, D.J. and Taylor, R.C.R. (1990) Local AIDS policies: planning and policy development for health promotion. *AIDS Progamme Paper* 6. London, Health Education Authority.

Cohen, D.R. and Henderson, J.B. (1988) *Health Prevention and Economics*. Oxford, Oxford University Press.

Cribb, A. and Haycox, A. (1989) Economic analysis and the evaluation of health promotion. *Community Medicine*, 11, 4, 299–305.

Drummond, M.F. (1980) *Principles of Economic Appraisal in Health Care*. Oxford, Oxford University Press.

Drummond, M.F., Stoddart, G.L. and Torrance, G.W. (1987) *Economic Evaluation of Health Care Programmes*. Oxford, Oxford University Press.

Engleman, S.R. and Forbes, J. (1984) *Economic Aspects of Health Education*. Occasional Paper No. 1, London, Health Education Council.

Godfrey, C., Hardman, G. and Maynard, A. (1989) *Priorities for Health Promotion: An Economic Approach*. Discussion Paper 59. York, University of York, Centre for Health Economics.

Guiguet, M. and Valleron, A.J. (1990) Demographic impact of mortality from AIDS in France: Projection for 1991. In D. Schwefel, R. Lendl, J. Rovira and M.F. Drummond (Eds.) *Economic Aspects of AIDS and HIV Infection*. Berlin, Springer-Verlag.

Harrison, L. and Tether, P. (1990) Information and voluntary agreements: the policy networks. In C. Godfrey and D. Robinson (Eds.) *Preventing Alcohol and Tobacco Problems Volume 2*. Aldershot, Avebury.

Maynard, A. (1990) The economic evaluation of care programmes for patients with HIV-AIDS. In D. Schwefel, R. Lendl, J. Rovira, and M.F. Drummond (Eds.) *Economic Aspects of AIDS and HIV Infection*. Berlin, Springer-Verlag

O'Brien, B.J. (1990) AIDS and subjective risk assessment: perspectives from the decision sciences. In M.F. Drummond and L.M. Davies (Eds.) *AIDS: The Challenge for Economic Analysis*. Birmingham, Health Services Management Centre.

PHLS (1990) *Acquired Immune Deficiency Syndrome in England and Wales to end of 1993: Projections using Data to end September 1989*. London, Public Health Laboratory Service.

Rees, M. (1990) AIDS/HIV costs in England: the case of the Oxfordshire District. In D. Schwefel, R. Lendl, J. Rovira and M.F. Drummond (Eds.) *Economic Aspects of AIDS and HIV Infection*. Berlin, Springer-Verlag.

Rovira, J. (1990a) Economic aspects of AIDS. In D. Schwefel, R. Lendl, J. Rovira and M.F. Drummond (Eds.) *Economic Aspects of AIDS and HIV Infection*. Berlin, Springer-Verlag.

Rovira J. (1990b) The economics of prevention. In M.F. Drummond and L.M. Davies (Eds.) *AIDS: The Challenge for Economic Analysis*. Birmingham, Health Services Management Centre.

Tolley, K. and Maynard, A. (1990) *Government Funding for Health and Social Care*. Forthcoming discussion paper. York, University of York, Centre for Health Economics.

Torrance, G. (1986) Measurement of health state utilities for economic appraisal. *Journal of Health Economics*, 5, 1, 1–30.

CHAPTER NINE

Challenges for the Nineties: Priorities and Needs in the Evaluation of HIV/AIDS Health Promotion

Andrea Young, Maryan Pye and Peter Aggleton

HIV/AIDS health promotion remains a relatively new and dynamic activity. This means that, while it is timely to consider different approaches to evaluation, there are also particular challenges posed by working in previously uncharted waters. Nevertheless, health education and health promotion workers see evaluation as an integral and necessary component of their work in a way which is possibly unique within the statutory services and the voluntary sector, and the challenges inherent in work with HIV/AIDS cannot be ignored.

In the field of treatment and care, progress tends to be made on the basis of what has been previously shown by others to be an acceptable intervention. For example, positive findings from randomised drug trials influence the practice of physicians and prescribers in a relatively straightforward manner. Once positive findings have been obtained, it is generally assumed that such interventions will have a benefit, so that any further evaluation is seen as an optional process, not to be embarked upon without additional resources. The accepted experience of others is therefore what influences the biomedical model of innovation. This is in marked contrast to the culture of health education and health promotion. Evaluation is seen here as a tool to assist in the planning, development and implementation of educational initiatives. It is integral to the process, and not a separate and easily transferable 'product'. Evaluation is therefore more commonly found as part of routine good practice – a conscious and deliberative process which guides and supports health promotion work.

The need to understand and demonstrate the effectiveness of health education and health promotion is especially felt by HIV/AIDS workers. There are many reasons and motives for evaluating HIV/ AIDS health education and health promotion, some of which have already been explored as part of the HEA's initiatives in local evaluation (see for example Pye and Kapila, 1990a). These are reflected in a demand by local workers and their managers for 'ready-made' approaches to evaluation (Moody *et al*, 1991). Yet there seems to be no readily accessible appropriate body of knowledge or experience to draw upon, a factor which only serves to heighten the problems of evaluating such work (Pye and Kapila, 1990b).

The consultation

In May 1990, the HEA, with the support of Bristol Polytechnic, convened a small group of experienced evaluators and local HIV/AIDS workers for a two-day consultation exercise. The purpose of the meeting was to share experiences, to discuss some of the specific problems and to begin to find ways in which local workers could best be supported in their evaluation work. At the consultation the evaluations described in the preceding chapters were presented. The activities which have been evaluated are typical of work in this field, in that they range from co-ordinated district-wide programmes to discrete individual interventions, such as theatre in education projects. Some of the contributions are more general in their approach, looking at activities such as training. Others examine innovative ways of evaluating specific HIV/AIDS health education and health promotion activities. Yet others describe styles of economic evaluation of a type that are not as yet fully developed in the health promotion field (Godfrey *et al*, 1989).

During the workshops and discussion groups that took place as part of the consultation, it became apparent that some local workers were unclear as to the extent to which they could adopt the approaches outlined by the academic experts. It was also clear that the term 'evaluation' meant quite different things to different people. Some of the local workers participating in the meeting provided accounts of the evaluation exercises which they had devised and undertaken, with apparent success in many cases. Despite this, doubts and uncertainties concerning the ability to undertake evaluation were frequently expressed. Many workers felt that they were insufficiently equipped with the necessary skills or training in research methods to be able to evaluate their work effectively. Workers also felt that evaluation should not be seen as an end in itself. Instead, it should be used to bring about improvements in their work. However, this demands a willingness to change on the part of managers and others who may find themselves in receipt of evaluation findings. Some workers spoke of the negative aspects of being asked to undertake evaluation without a clear rationale or plan, or of producing reports which were prepared to satisfy funders or managers, but which were then merely shelved. Often, sponsors' and managers' hopes from evaluation were considered unrealistic, because they in fact held unrealistic expectations of what a particular project or initiative could achieve (e.g. in delivering behaviour change). This underlined the importance of identifying and defining in advance the aims and objectives of the evaluation, together with an agreed definition as to what will count as success.

Earlier chapters detailing the experience of independent evaluations in Cambridge (Chapter three) and Manchester (Chapter four) have confirmed the need for a prior commitment to respond to evaluation findings. They also highlighted how evaluation is an interactive process, one which inevitably inflluences the work of the programme in some way. Local HIV/AIDS workers observed that this influence could operate at many levels, since evaluation might easily interrupt the spontaneity of an educational initiative or, at the very least, divert some of the available resources for HIV/AIDS health education and health promotion. However, if the evaluation was genuinely participatory and not simply used as a mechanical tool, it was possible to change a project's direction or objectives. This could be constructive and reinforced the need to assess both processes and outcomes in evaluation.

Workers were also keen to explore the possible motives for evaluation, since some of these motives were felt to influence the answers obtained in evaluation exercises, if not the kinds of questions asked. Evaluation was seen as offering a valuable opportunity for critical assessment of one's own work. This was recognised as a positive aspect, and one which encouraged personal and professional development through informed practice. Other motives for evaluation included:

- to satisfy management pressures
- to meet budgetary or funding considerations
- to enhance team building
- to inform the programme or project
- to wield political influence
- to influence policy development.

However, no one approach to evaluation was considered likely to meet all these needs, or to satisfy all interested parties. Each of the stakeholders in evaluation – including the workers, managers, funders, the community or recipients – was felt to have different interests. In particular, the requirement from managers or funders to evaluate in terms of narrowly defined, quantifiable outcomes was a source of constant frustration. It was felt that managers did not have sufficient grasp of the contexts in which local HIV/AIDS health education and health promotion takes place to be able to interpret such information in a meaningful way.

On the positive side, evaluation could be used by local workers to validate new or radical ways of working. It could also demonstrate good practice in HIV/AIDS health promotion. In order to share findings with others in the field it was considered necessary that evaluation data should be generalisable and not too specific. This could be relatively easy when monitoring levels of activity, but was more difficult when it came to accounting for what actually happened as part of a health education or health promotion activity. Identifying appropriate indicators to examine these issues posed a particular challenge.

Various types of evaluation were identified as important by health educators. The relevance of evaluating the process of HIV/AIDS health promotion was recognised, but there was also an enthusiasm to investigate effectiveness by comparing outcomes with the aims and objectives of individual initiatives. Most workers felt constrained by a lack of human and financial resources and were also concerned with cost-effectiveness in assessing whether planned initiatives had met the community's or participants' needs. It was also pointed out that there was little point in amassing reams of evaluation data if there was not the time to analyse it or to consider its possible impact on future programme development.

Evaluations which sought to consider the impact of particular initiatives on self-empowerment, healthy decision-making and behaviour change were considered highly relevant, but posed quite different problems for local workers. This was especially true when an initiative had taken place in an informal setting (e.g. outreach work with homeless young people), where it was hard to maintain contact with the client group, and where there were problems in isolating the relevant source of influence. In these instances there was a tendency simply to monitor levels of activity rather than to attempt to define and measure outcomes.

Clearly, some aspects of HIV/AIDS health education and health promotion were felt to be more amenable to simple evaluation techniques than others. Training initiatives were most frequently cited, with evaluation being undertaken through self-completed pre-and post-course questionnaires, and occasional follow-up interviews. However, it was questioned whether workers needed to evaluate the same training courses every time. Was evaluation here concerned with monitoring the trainer's performance on each occasion, or with assessing the relevance and suitability of the course? If the latter was the case, then surely 'one-off' evaluation might be more appropriate, bearing in mind earlier considerations of staff resources.

Discussion also took place concerning who or what should be the legitimate focus of evaluation, and from whose viewpoint could an initiative be described as a success. Key stakeholders here could include the workers or service deliverers, the evaluators, the managers or the recipients. Evaluation findings could vary enormously depending upon who answered the questions. An example was given by one trainer, who described an HIV/AIDS awareness training session in which participants rejected the notion of personal risk in relation to HIV transmission but asked for more information about risks from health care practices (risks that are statistically almost negligible). Had such an initiative, which was deemed by the recipients as not meeting their needs, necessarily failed? These experiences highlighted some of the different levels at which evaluation could operate, as well as the difficulties experienced in trying to elicit the 'truth' about what happened in circumstances where there may be differing interpretations of what went on.

There were also felt to be problems in striving to be objective when evaluating one's own work. It was difficult to disentangle personal assumptions and values from those of the project or initiative when trying to examine critically what might be appropriate or useful. The local worker was likely to be aware of nuances within, and influences upon, an initiative which an external evaluator might not detect. This should not always be seen as an obstacle to good evaluation. Some workers felt that honesty was a better approach than striving to attain a possibly spurious sense of accuracy or objectivity.

Throughout the consultation there were expressions of concern about apparently conflicting views and approaches. Different views were often expressed about whether evaluation should best be internal or external, qualitative or quantitative, subjective or objective, a worker's tool or a something to be used by managers. These polarised points of view often served to make aspects of evaluation seem inaccessible and unacceptable to local workers. Through further exploration of these issues it may be possible to reconcile some of the unhelpful differences.

Reconciling the differences

Participants in the consultation tended to view external evaluators as the 'experts' – people who were highly skilled, objective (by virtue of their externality) and with the time and resources to undertake the work in a professional manner. In contrast, in-house evaluation was often associated with a lack of skills, time and funds. However, there can be negative aspects to external evaluation, especially when it is experienced as intrusive or disruptive to a programme. Both internal and external evaluation can suffer when the process is seen as time-consuming or a source of pressure, anxiety or misunderstanding.

In preceding chapters, Sue Scott (Chapter four) and Alan Prout (Chapter five), in the role of external evaluators, advocate a participatory or broadly ethnographic approach to evaluation. They argue that it is only by getting into the programme that the evaluator can focus on questions of real interest to the stakeholders. By doing this, an external evaluator can become more aware of the context in which the activity is taking place, the energy and commitment of the workers, and the stress and pressures that can affect certain actions or decisions. The evaluator should be both observant and involved, otherwise there is the risk of missing out important details. Evaluation should aim to be reflexive, in that it develops according to the situation and the context, consonant with the notion of interactive process. These authors therefore reject the idea that evaluation can proceed outside of an initiative, as a static and discrete activity. Such an approach argues that, regardless of whether the evaluator is internal or external to the programme, broadly similar techniques need to be adopted in order to generate meaningful and valid feedback.

Local workers are acutely aware of the pressure to generate quantitative data and measurable outcomes. These are seen as carrying greater weight and status with managers. Taken in isolation, however, quantitative data are often felt to lack meaning and validity. For example, an evaluation process which simply monitors levels of activity will not indicate why these levels might fluctuate and what the factors are that might influence them. There is a general wariness among HIV/AIDS workers about the possibility that quantitative data can all too easily be lifted out of its original context and be misinterpreted, or used in a negative way.

In his chapter on the evaluation of a syringe and needle exchange scheme, Graham Hart describes the limitations of adopting a traditional public health/epidemiological approach to evaluation which defines success solely in terms of a fall in the number of new infections (Chapter seven). This is particularly problematic in the field of HIV/AIDS, where the persistent stigma and discrimination surrounding known HIV status mean that we can interpret accurately very little about the spread of the epidemic from HIV-antibody test reports. Hart emphasises how qualitative information is critical in contextualising quantitative data in order to make sense of why attendance at the syringe and needle exchange fluctuated.

As Hart points out, service providers were interested in different and more easily quantifiable outcomes, such as the numbers of people attracted into the service, the number of contacts maintained and the number of clients who went on to gain access to other forms of health education. Evaluators and project workers, on the other hand, were concerned to learn more about the drug-using practices and behaviour of clients, in order that they could match service provision more appropriately to client needs. However, the evaluators did not have a remit to carry through this work. This highlights the problems of an evaluation brief being set to serve the needs of those other than the workers or service providers.

Even within the most obviously quantitative approach, there is a recognition of the place for qualitative input. In describing the work of health economists, for example, Christine Godfrey and Keith Tolley argue that, in assessing the effects of HIV/AIDS health education, both health care costs and social costs need to be borne in mind (Chapter eight). The latter might include the effects of discrimination on the ability of people with AIDS to live in the community or to keep working. These phenomena are not readily enumerated but rely on qualitative understanding and value-laden assumptions. These authors therefore suggest that successful evaluation will rely upon both kinds of data. Quantitative and qualitative data are not seen in direct opposition to one another, but rather as complementary partners which are mutually supporting and reinforcing.

Similar issues can arise in debates about whether evaluation should be objective or subjective. Objectivity is often seen as having high premium and being all-important. Subjectivity is considered by many to be a flaw in evaluation; local workers identify it as a weakness, yet it is often felt to be unavoidable. Several of the contributing authors, in their role as external evaluators, spoke of bringing their own professional and personal backgrounds and expertise to the evaluation exercises with which they had been associated. This was felt to be a valuable asset which need not detract from the authenticity or validity of the work with which they were involved. A balance had to be struck between objectivity (which may overlook the real meaning of what is happening) and subjectivity (which may be accused of bias). This tension is perhaps best exemplified in the model outlined by Robert McEwan and Rajinder Bhopal (Chapter two), who suggest that optimal results may be obtained by combining elements of subjective and objective evaluation. This does not preclude the evaluation from being a disciplined activity. Rather, it can make the process more flexible and can lead to the evaluation of all aspects of a programme or initiative, including its implementation, its impact, its acceptability and its efficiency.

David Armstrong and Jean Hutton in their examination of a systemic model for evaluating HIV/AIDS health promotion programmes (Chapter three) emphasise the importance of bringing what they describe as the 'whole system' into view. They argue that evaluation needs to focus both on processes and on outcomes before making connections between the two. The key question to be asked is, 'What is making something happen?' Answering this necessarily involves getting into the programme and drawing upon subjective knowledge to interpret and make sense of the links. Some of these links may become more apparent as the evaluator identifies the programme's outputs. These are often more visible than outcomes, at least in the short to medium term.

Evaluation should not be too narrowly defined, as long-term or unintended outcomes may be lost. By concentrating solely on outcomes one cannot make good practice explicit, nor account for why certain expected outcomes may not be achieved. As HIV/AIDS health education and health promotion programmes are dynamic and susceptible to change, these changes need to be accounted for in the evaluation process, because they may impact upon the outcome. Evaluation therefore needs to concentrate both on processes and on outcomes if it is to be either informative or useful.

Evaluators and their funders or managers need to discuss and negotiate the purpose, approach, content and timing of evaluation. Workers and managers should also satisfy themselves that the information they are seeking can be used constructively afterwards. It is important to agree beforehand on the criteria or indicators that will be used to assess effectiveness, as these can be a source of conflict. Evaluation reports should be written in an appropriate format which presents relevant information in a readable style. There needs to be a pre-existing commitment to receiving and discussing evaluation reports and to using their findings in planning future activities or directions.

Throughout the consultation, the view emerged that the best kinds of evaluation were those that were eclectic rather than narrowly focused. In reality there are no ready-made answers, nor is there one right way in which to evaluate. The preceding chapters illustrate some of the potential pitfalls or critical issues to consider; they do not offer a definitive guide to evaluation. The choice of approach needs to be based upon questions relating to the nature and objectives of the activity under study, and it needs to draw upon the methods that are most appropriate and useful to the issue in hand.

The way forward

In the final session of the consultation, participants brought together some suggestions about how the evaluation of HIV/AIDS health education and health promotion could be further developed. A theme common to all was the need to demystify the functions, processes and language of evaluation so as to make it more accessible to workers who did not see themselves as experts.

Networks were also needed at both national and local levels. Nationally, it was hoped that a resource directory of existing projects might be put together to disseminate examples of good practice. The production of this could be facilitated by a national body such as the HEA through the medium of its Inter-Regional HIV/AIDS Forum, or through publications such as *AIDS Dialogue*. A regularly updated section on evaluation might also prove a useful supplement to the

National AIDS Manual. Evaluation should also become a routine agenda item to be discussed at all seminars and conferences.

Local networks could provide opportunities to pool expertise and to share 'hands-on' experience. It was accepted that there were often unrecognised local sources of expertise to draw upon, and one function of local networks could be to establish more effective links between HIV/AIDS health educators and health promoters and relevant academic departments in polytechnics, universities and medical schools.

The need was expressed for a resource pack which would provide a basic jargon-free guide to evaluation methodology. This should offer a step-by-step guide to identifying an appropriate approach, clarifying the evaluation questions to be asked and identifying new methods. It should also offer some 'off the peg' solutions to familiar evaluation problems. To support this, a programme of training in evaluation skills would be needed. The emphasis here would be on applying theory to the solving of practical problems, thereby building a bridge between 'academic' and 'pragmatic' approaches. An HEA training programme and an evaluation manual (Aggleton *et al,* 1992) are in fact forthcoming.

Finally, it was suggested that other stakeholders who had an interest in evaluation (managers, sponsors, funders) needed educating about the advantages and disadvantages of various approaches, the limitations and pitfalls of an undue dependence on health outcome measures and performance indicators, the need for adequate resourcing when evaluation is set up, and the need for a prior commitment to respond to evaluation findings.

The broader context

Given the clarity with which these needs were identified, it is important by way of conclusion to explore and expand on the ideas expressed in the light of the prevailing political climate around HIV/AIDS and health promotion as they relate to current priorities in the health and social services.

The establishment of the HEA in 1987 to lead the national effort to limit the epidemic of HIV infection marked the recognition by government of the importance of health education in achieving this aim. It was followed by financial commitment over successive years with earmarked funding to support a range of complementary health promotion initiatives at a local level. Now, in the early 1990s, it is possible that the high point for funding for HIV/AIDS education may soon pass. The downward revision of short-term projections of the epidemic has been widely misunderstood, and irresponsible elements of the media have erroneously promoted the notion that there is negligible risk associated with unprotected heterosexual sex.

At the same time, political energies have been diverted to implementing the changes in the health service which arise from the government's White Papers on hospital, community and primary care services. However, the philosophy which underlies these changes does provide opportunities to further develop work in HIV/AIDS health promotion. It has, for example, been restated explicitly that the National Health Service has responsibility to promote health and prevent disease. These functions are no longer to be seen as an optional extra at the expense of services for treatment or care. The philosophy of a service based on negotiated contracts also introduces the need to specify quality and to implement arrangements for monitoring based on the measurement of outputs and outcomes, in terms of both quality and quantity.

Many of the proposals put forward in this book in relation to the evaluation of HIV/AIDS health promotion are applicable to the broader field of health education and health promotion. The new emphasis on 'value for money' will increasingly call for a health economist's view when it comes to making choices. Health promotion evaluation will also have to develop measures to value the resources consumed, and the benefits attained, if it is to obtain or justify the continued allocation of funds. Reliable and rapid appraisal techniques are needed which are capable of producing timely results in clear and accessible form to feed into the contracting process. Much of what has been learned so far about HIV/AIDS health promotion relates to the processes it involves (Pye and Kapila, 1990b); increasingly, there is likely to be a demand for measures of intermediate outputs and overall health outcomes in order to assess the quality and quantity of service contract activity in the new-look National Health Service.

It will become increasingly necessary for health educators and health promoters to disseminate more widely findings from the evaluations with which they are associated. In the clinical field and in mainstream education, established networks of professional meetings and journals are often used to disseminate findings from research and evaluation activity. Once subjected to peer review in this way, these findings may be accepted into, or rejected from, the recognised body of knowledge within these fields. Advances in health education and health promotion methodology should be subject to the same critical scrutiny and communicated through a parallel set of channels.

The 1990s offer a unique set of challenges for HIV/AIDS health education and health promotion. Management structures are adapting in response to the emergence of purchaser and provider roles within the health and social services. HIV/AIDS work is increasingly being 'normalised' to take its place alongside other activities. The time is now ripe for aspects of HIV/AIDS work to be integrated into the mainstream of health promotion, and for generic health education/ promotion professionals to learn from the experience of their more specialised colleagues. While the focus may be distinctive, the general principles involved in monitoring and evaluating HIV/AIDS work are not new. There is, therefore, much to be gained from working closely with those who already have experience of the techniques involved and the strategies needed to implement them.

References

Aggleton, P.J., Moody, D. and Young, A. (1992). *Evaluating HIV/AIDS Health Promotion: A resource for HIV/AIDS health promotion workers in statutory and voluntary organisations.* London, Health Education Authority.

Godfrey, C., Hardman, G. and Maynard, A. (1989). *Priorities for Health Promotion.* Discussion Paper 59. York, University of York, Centre for Health Economics.

Moody, D., Aggleton, P., Kapila, M., Pye, M. and Young, A. (1991) Monitoring and evaluating local HIV/AIDS health promotion: a review of theory and practice. *HIV/ AIDS & Sexual Health Programme Paper 11.* London, Health Education Authority.

Pye, M. and Kapila, M. (1990a). Evaluation of AIDS health promotion programmes: concepts and the Cambridge study. *HIV/AIDS & Sexual Health Programme Paper 7.* London, Health Education Authority.

Pye, M. and Kapila, M. (1990b). The story so far . . . a review of the evaluation of local AIDS programmes. *HIV/AIDS & Sexual Health Programme Paper 9.* London, Health Education Authority.

Contributors

Peter Aggleton is Director of the Health and Education Research Unit in the Faculty of Education, Goldsmiths' College, University of London. He manages a number of major projects concerned with HIV/AIDS health promotion. His recent publications include *Nursing Models and the Nursing Process* (with Helen Chalmers, Macmillan, 1986). *Deviance* (Tavistock, 1987), *Social Aspects of AIDS* (ed. with Hilary Homans, Falmer, 1988), *AIDS: Social Representations, Social Practices* (ed. with Graham Hart and Peter Davies, Falmer, 1989), *AIDS: Scientific and Social Issues* (with Hilary Homans, Jan Mojsa, Stuart Watson and Simon Watney, Churchill Livingstone, 1989), *Health* (Routledge, 1990), *AIDS: Individual, Cultural and Policy Dimensions* (ed. with Peter Davies and Graham Hart, Falmer, 1990) and *AIDS: Responses, Interventions and Care* (ed. with Peter Davies and Graham Hart, Falmer, 1991).

David Armstrong is a director of the Grubb Institute, London. His research interests are organisational analysis within systemic and psychoanalytic frames of reference. He works across the Grubb Institute's programme of applied research and consultancy in industry and commerce, health and social services, education, criminal justice agencies, voluntary organisations and churches. Recent publications include *Ensuring the Future – Evaluation of the Cambridge AIDS Programme* (with Jean Hutton, Grubb Institute, 1989) and *Evaluating AIDS Health Promotion Programmes – A Model for Local Organisational Initiatives* (with Jean Hutton, Grubb Institute, 1989).

Rajinder Bhopal is Senior Lecturer and Consultant in Public Health Medicine at the University of Newcastle upon Tyne. He has a broad range of research interests in epidemiology and health service research. Recent work on HIV/AIDS includes evaluation research and monitoring the HIV/AIDS epidemic in the Northern Region.

Wendy Clark is a freelance training and development consultant working predominantly in the areas of organisational change and management development. She has been involved in HIV/AIDS work for many years in a voluntary and professional capacity. Her activities include training and development, policy formulation, evaluation and consultancy support to HIV/AIDS projects. She is the author of a *Training Handbook on HIV/AIDS for Local Authorities* (HEA/LGTB, 1989) and is currently working on two other complementary publications for the Health Education Authority.

Christine Godfrey is a Research Fellow at the Centre for Health Economics, University of York. Her research interests include the economic evaluation of health education/promotion activities, and she is Co-director of a joint project with the Health Education Authority on cost-effectiveness in health promotion. She is the co-editor of *Quality of Life: Perspectives and Policies* (with Sally Baldwin and Carol Propper, Routledge, 1990) and *Preventing Alcohol and Tobacco Problems Volume 2* (with David Robinson, Avebury, 1990).

Graham Hart is Lecturer in Medical Sociology at University College and Middlesex School of Medicine, London. His research interests include sexual and injecting risk behaviours for HIV infection, and he has recently published papers on these subjects in the *British Medical Journal*, *AIDS* and *AIDS Care*. He is the editor (with Peter Aggleton and Peter Davies) of *AIDS: Social Representations, Social Practices* (Falmer, 1989), *AIDS: Individual, Cultural and Policy Dimensions* (Falmer, 1990) and *AIDS: Responses, Interventions and Care* (Falmer, 1991).

Jean Hutton is a director of the Grubb Institute, London and of the Institute's Centre for Explorations in Social Concern. She works on organisational analysis, management and leadership in institutions in the UK and overseas. Current research interests include the human and social implications of HIV/AIDS, school-generated management and community mediation schemes. Her recent publications include *Ensuring the Future – Evaluation of the Cambridge AIDS Programme* (with David Armstrong, Grubb Institute, 1989), *Evaluating AIDS Health Promotion Programmes – A Model for Local Organisational Initiatives* (with David Armstrong, Grubb Institute, 1989) and *Thinking about AIDS* (Centre for Explorations in Social Concern/Grubb Institute, 1989).

Mukesh Kapila was the Deputy Director of the AIDS Programme at the Health Education Authority between 1987 and 1990. He has spoken and written extensively on AIDS and other international public health issues, and served frequently as an Adviser to the World Health Organisation and other bodies. He was responsible for initiating the HEA's Local AIDS Programme Evaluation Support Initiative, on which this book is based. He is now Senior Health and Population Adviser to the Overseas Development Administration in the UK Foreign and Commonwealth Office.

Robert McEwan is a research associate in the Division of Community Medicine at the University of Newcastle upon Tyne. His main research interest is in the evaluation of preventive health care progammes. He is currently completing a PhD evaluating a health screening programme for elderly people.

Diane Moody was a research associate on the HEA-funded HIV/AIDS Local Evaluation Support Project at Bristol Polytechnic. She is the co-author (with Peter Aggleton, Mukesh Kapila, Maryan Pye and Andrea Young) of *Monitoring and Evaluating Local HIV/AIDS Health Education and Health Promotion Programmes, HIV/AIDS & Sexual Health Programme Paper 11* (HEA).

Alan Prout is a medical sociologist and Director of the MSc in Medical Social Anthropology at the University of Keele. Previously a researcher at Cambridge University and a teacher at South Bank Polytechnic, he has carried out a number of research proiects related to health education. He is currently an evaluator on the MESMAC Project.

Maryan Pye is Professional Adviser to Cambridgeshire Family Health Services Authority. Between 1988 and 1990 she was Special Adviser to the HEA's AIDS Programme. She has enduring interests in health education and health promotion.

Sue Scott is Lecturer in Sociology at the University of Manchester. She is a member of the Women, Risk and AIDS Project (WRAP) team and Director of the Centre for Research into Social Aspects of Health (CRISAH). Her research and teaching interests are in the sociology of health, sexuality and research methodology. She is currently writing a book entitled *Feminist Researching* for Routledge.

Keith Tolley is a research fellow at the Centre for Health Economics, University of York. He is currently involved in research into the economics of social care for people with HIV infection or AIDS.

Andrea Young was formerly an AIDS programme officer and is now the Policy Development Officer, Public Health Division, at the Health Education Authority, London. She remains the project officer responsible for the HEA's Local AIDS Programme Evaluation Support Initiative.